EVIDENCE-BASED MEDICINE: 500 CLUES TO DIAGNOSIS AND TREATMENT

D0879507

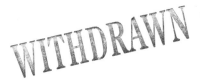

EVIDENCE-BASED MEDICINE: 500 CLUES TO DIAGNOSIS AND TREATMENT

Todd B. Ellerin, M.D.
Senior Assistant Resident
Osler Medical Service
Department of Internal Medicine
Johns Hopkins University School of Medicine
Baltimore, Maryland

Luis A. Diaz, Jr., M.D.
Senior Assistant Resident
Osler Medical Service
Department of Internal Medicine
Johns Hopkins University School of Medicine
Baltimore, Maryland

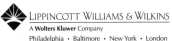

LIPPINCOTT WILLIAMS & WILKINS
A **Wolters Kluwer** Company
Philadelphia · Baltimore · New York · London
Buenos Aires · Hong Kong · Sydney · Tokyo

BS

Acquisitions Editor: Richard Winters
Developmental Editor: Lisa Consoli
Production Editor: Emily Lerman
Manufacturing Manager: Benjamin Rivera
Cover Designer: Christine Jenny
Compositor: Circle Graphics
Printer: Victor Graphics

© 2001 by LIPPINCOTT WILLIAMS & WILKINS
530 Walnut Street
Philadelphia, PA 19106 USA
LWW.com

Printed in the USA

Library of Congress Cataloging-in-Publication Data

Ellerin, Todd B.
    Evidence-based medicine: 500 clues to diagnosis and treatment / authors, Todd B. Ellerin, Luis A. Diaz, Jr.
      p. ; cm.
    Includes bibliographical references and index.
    ISBN 0-7817-3280-8
    1. Internal medicine—Case studies. 2. Diagnosis—Case studies.
3. Evidence-based medicine. I. Diaz, Luis A. II. Title.
    [DNLM: 1. Diagnostic Techniques and Procedures—Case Report.
2. Diagnostic Techniques and Procedures—Problems and Exercises.
3. Evidence-Based Medicine—methods—Case Report. 4. Evidence-Based Medicine—methods—Problems and Exercises. 5. Internal Medicine—methods—Case Report. 6. Internal Medicine—methods—Problems and Exercises. WB 18.2 E45e 2001]
RC66 .E45 2001
616—dc21

2001016486

9/8/04

10 9 8 7 6 5 4 3 2 1

To my parents, Barbara and Phil, and to the rest of my family
for their enormous support
and to my teachers and colleagues
who are a continuous source of inspiration.

—TBE

To my parents for their love and guidance
and to Michele and Jacob
for reminding me what is truly important.

—LAD

Note

The nonpossessive form for eponyms is used throughout this text, in accordance with the commentary by Victor A. McKusick, M.D. [McKusick VA. On the naming of clinical disorders, with particular reference to eponyms. *Medicine* 1998; 77(1):1–2].

CONTENTS

REVIEWERS

John G. Bartlett, M.D.
Chief, Division of Infectious Diseases and Professor of Medicine, Johns Hopkins University School of Medicine, Baltimore, Maryland

Edward J. Benz, Jr., M.D.
President, Dana Farber Cancer Institute; Professor of Medicine, Harvard Medical School, Boston, Massachusetts

Michael J. Choi, M.D.
Assistant Professor of Medicine, Division of Nephrology, Johns Hopkins University School of Medicine, Baltimore, Maryland

Ross Donehower, M.D.
Director, Oncology Fellowship Program and Professor of Medicine, Department of Oncology, Johns Hopkins University School of Medicine, Baltimore, Maryland

Joel E. Gallant, M.D., M.P.H.
Medical Director, Johns Hopkins Moore Clinic; Associate Professor of Medicine, Division of Infectious Diseases, Johns Hopkins University School of Medicine, Baltimore, Maryland

David B. Hellmann, M.D., F.A.C.P.
Chairman, Department of Medicine, Johns Hopkins Bayview Medical Center; Mary Betty Stevens Professor of Medicine, Johns Hopkins University School of Medicine, Baltimore, Maryland

FOREWORD

I am very grateful to the wise mentor who many years ago advised me to try to learn one lesson from each patient that I evaluated. Medicine, he realized, was too vast and ever-changing to be mastered quickly. Therefore, learning one lesson from each patient became my mantra for the interns and residents who have served on the Osler Medical Service of the Johns Hopkins Hospital over the last 14 years. One of the teaching conferences that best reinforced this philosophy of learning was afternoon report, where the residents would present to each other the most instructive patients admitted to the hospital or evaluated in the clinics. At this conference, and many others, the residents would often emphasize the main teaching point by reviewing a pertinent article from the medical literature. Drs. Diaz and Ellerin have gone several steps further by collecting and distilling the most useful clinical lessons from all the teaching conferences throughout Johns Hopkins Hospital into this attractive book of medical pearls. In crafting this book, they have chosen clues from all fields of medicine, have reviewed the clues with faculty experts, and, wherever possible, have certified the value of each clue with a reference. The end result is a terrific book that will make learning important lessons from patients easy and enjoyable for medical students, residents, and attending physicians. I believe readers will join me in applauding Drs. Ellerin and Diaz for their scholarship.

David B. Hellmann, M.D.
Mary Betty Stevens Professor of Medicine
Johns Hopkins University School of Medicine
Baltimore, Maryland

PREFACE

Morning report is often cited as a favorite conference among house officers. One reason is that we are challenged with unknown diagnostic dilemmas and charged with the responsibility of solving them. In one sense, we need to be medical detectives. How can we learn to be better diagnosticians? Experience is an essential ingredient, but it is impossible to have twenty years of patient care under one's belt as an intern fresh out of medical school. Secondly, a strong knowledge base empowers the clinician to think critically and solve medical mysteries. Lastly, heuristics, or short cuts, are often used by master clinicians to simplify complex medical cases and arrive at correct diagnoses.

Evidence-Based Medicine: 500 Clues to Diagnosis and Treatment has been written, by medicine residents, specifically to promulgate relevant medical heuristics. This book is targeted to medical detectives. It focuses on patient-oriented diagnostic dilemmas, differential diagnoses, pathognomonic sign-and-symptom complexes, and shortcuts to problem solving. We use the term "clue" to signify critical medical information passed down from expert clinicians to improve patient care, enhance diagnostic acumen, and facilitate patient work-ups. These clues are not original. Many have been uttered on morning rounds for years, signifying that they have withstood the test of time. We provide representative references for these clues in our era of evidence-based medicine. These clues are patient-oriented and will be most helpful by the bedside—the place where most answers in medicine are found.

Good Luck.

Todd B. Ellerin, M.D.
Luis A. Diaz, Jr., M.D.

ACKNOWLEDGMENTS

We acknowledge the members of the Osler medical service, particularly the Barker Firm. To David B. Hellmann, M.D., John J. Mann, M.D., Victor A. McKusick, M.D., and Charlie M. Wiener, M.D., for their example as dedicated teachers, physicians, and leaders. We extend a special thanks to our reviewers and especially to Richard Winters from Lippincott Williams & Wilkins for his ongoing support. Finally, and most importantly, to our patients, who continue to teach us every day.

AIDS/HIV

1. The two most likely causes of the **human immuno-deficiency virus (HIV)-associated cholangiopathy** are cytomegalovirus (CMV) and cryptosporidiosis. This disease should be considered in a patient infected with HIV with right upper quadrant abdominal pain and a rising alkaline phosphatase. Endoscopic retrograde cholangiopancreatography commonly demonstrates papillary stenosis (1,2).

2. In a patient infected with HIV who presents with shortness of breath, the presence of a pleural effusion on chest x-ray (CXR) study makes *Pneumocystis carinii* **pneumonia (PCP)** less likely, and should prompt an alternative diagnosis (3).

3. The most common infectious cause of **cauda equina syndrome** in an HIV-infected patient with a CD4 count less than 50 cells/mm^3 is CMV (4).

4. The most common cause of **fever of unknown origin** in patients with acquired immunodeficiency syndrome (AIDS) in many case series is *Mycobacterium avium* complex (MAC) (5).

5. The presence of an **osteolytic** lesion in a patient infected with HIV who has a CD4 count less than 200 cells/mm^3 should raise suspicion for bartonellosis (agent of cat scratch disease and bacillary angiomatosis) (6).

6. Single or multiple **central nervous system (CNS) mass lesions** in an HIV-infected patient suggests three diagnoses: toxoplasmosis, primary CNS lymphoma, and progressive multifocal leukoencephalopathy (PML). Patients with negative anti-*Toxoplasma* IgG

titers are less likely to have toxoplasmosis, but a negative serology does not exclude the diagnosis. On imaging with magnetic resonance imaging (MRI), toxoplasmosis and lymphoma both enhance with contrast in contradistinction to PML. PML, usually limited to the white matter, is associated with a positive JC virus polymerase chain reaction (PCR) in the cerebrospinal fluid, whereas primary CNS lymphoma is associated with a positive Epstein-Barr virus (EBV) PCR (7–9).

7. Consider **parvovirus B19** in an HIV-infected patient with an isolated chronic anemia of unknown origin, especially when the reticulocyte count approaches zero (10,11).

8. If PCP is suspected, the workup should not end with a negative induced-sputum. This test is not sensitive enough to exclude PCP. A **bronchoscopy with bronchoalveolar lavage** should be pursued, as it has a sensitivity >95% (12,13).

9. In intravenous heroin abusers infected with HIV who present with renal insufficiency and proteinuria, it is often necessary to differentiate between **heroin nephropathy** and **HIV-associated nephropathy (HIVAN)**. These two entities differ with respect to the rate of progression: Heroin nephropathy is an indolent disease that typically leads to ESRD over a period of years. HIVAN, on the other hand, can lead to ESRD within a period of weeks to months. On renal ultrasound, the kidneys are diminished in size in heroin nephropathy, whereas the kidneys maintain their size in HIVAN. Renal biopsy may reveal focal segmental glomerulosclerosis in both conditions; however, the FSGS of HIVAN has a characteristic collapsing appearance (14–17).

10. **Cutaneous cryptococcosis** in a patient infected with HIV can be clinically indistinguishable from the umbilicated papules of molluscum contagiosum. The diagnosis can be made from biopsy of the "molluscum-like" lesions (18).

11. Most patients who present with **HIVAN** (focal segmental glomerulosclerosis) are black. Although nephrotic

range proteinuria is common, hypertension and edema occur in a minority of patients. IgA nephropathy is much less common and has only been reported in white patients (19,20).

12. PCP in a patient infected with HIV who is on **aerosolized pentamidine prophylaxis** has a predilection for the lung apices and extrapulmonary sites. These are uncommon presentations for classic PCP, which predominantly affects the perihilar zones and bases (21,22).

13. A patient infected with HIV who has a CD4 count less than 200 cells/mm^3 who presents with dyspnea on exertion and interstitial infiltrates on CXR is less likely to have PCP if the lactate dehydrogenase (LDH) is normal. LDH is a sensitive, but nonspecific marker for PCP (23).

14. **Spontaneous pneumothorax** in a patient infected with HIV is caused by PCP until proved otherwise, and empiric treatment should be initiated (24).

15. The most common infectious cause of an acute abdomen in a patient with AIDS and a CD4 count less than 50 cells/mm^3 is **CMV colitis** (25).

16. Bloody diarrhea is not a clinical feature of **disseminated MAC** in patients with AIDS. Watery diarrhea is more common (26,27).

17. **Disseminated histoplasmosis** is more common in patients with AIDS than in immunocompetent hosts. Features include fever, anorexia, weight loss, hepatosplenomegaly, pancytopenia, and sepsis. Bone marrow examination has significant diagnostic yield for isolating *Histoplasmosis capsulatum* and should be pursued early in the workup of disseminated histoplasmosis. Other assays used to detect the presence of this fungus are serum and urine *H. capsulatum* polysaccharide antigen (28–30).

18. A patient infected with HIV who presents with dysphagia and oral thrush has a high probability of having **esophageal candidiasis** and should be empirically treated. However, approximately 20% of such patients

who present with esophageal candidiasis will have no evidence of oral thrush. Focal odynophagia makes esophageal candidiasis less likely and ulcerative esophagitis the more likely culprit. Causes of esophageal ulcers include herpes simplex virus, CMV, and aphthous esophagitis. Lack of response to empiric antifungal therapy is an indication for diagnostic endoscopy (31,32).

19. The antiretroviral medications that cause **peripheral neuropathy** begin with the letter "d": ddC (zalcitabine), ddI (didanosine), and d4T (stavudine) (33).

20. *Cryptococcus neoformans* is the most common cause of **meningitis** in patients with AIDS who have CD4 counts less than 100 cells/mm³. Patients rarely present with the complete meningitis triad. The serum cryptococcal antigen is a highly sensitive screening test; when positive, it should always be followed by a lumbar puncture (34,35).

21. Systemic **non-Hodgkin lymphoma (NHL)** in a patient infected with HIV does not commonly present with generalized superficial lymphadenopathy, but rather as extranodal disease. The most common site of presentation is the gastrointestinal tract. Although uncommon, NHL can involve the lungs, presenting either with multiple pulmonary nodules or diffuse interstitial infiltrates. Most cases are associated with pleural effusions with or without concomitant parenchymal involvement. This is important clinically, because it can be distinguished from the pleural effusion associated with **Kaposi sarcoma**, which does not occur as an isolated effusion, but rather as an effusion with adjacent parenchymal abnormality (36,37).

22. **CMV polyradiculopathy** should be suspected in a patient with a CD4 count less than 50 cells/mm³ who presents with progressive lower extremity weakness, decreased lower extremity reflexes, urinary retention, and spinal cord imaging demonstrating thickening of the cauda equina. A lumbar puncture typically demonstrates a pronounced polymorphonuclear pleocytosis and a positive CMV PCR (38,39).

23. **Disseminated MAC** should be considered in any febrile patient with a CD4 count less than 50 cells/mm³. The patient may also present with abdominal pain, weight loss, anorexia, and watery diarrhea. Abdominal computed tomography scan may demonstrate hepatosplenomegaly and mesenteric adenopathy. Empiric therapy is rarely necessary: The diagnosis is made definitively by positive mycobacterial blood cultures (40,41).

24. The patient infected with HIV presenting to the emergency room with tachypnea, dyspnea, abdominal pain, and an anion gap metabolic acidosis should be tested for **nucleoside analog-induced lactic acidosis**. Laboratory abnormalities include low serum bicarbonate, elevated serum lactate, elevated aminotransferases, and elevated creatine kinase. Abdominal CT scan often shows fatty infiltration of the liver. This syndrome is thought to be a result of mitochondrial toxicity. Cases have been reported of simultaneous presentation of nucleoside-induced pancreatitis and lactic acidosis in patients with AIDS (42–44).

25. **Acute retroviral syndrome** (primary HIV infection) can present like mononucleosis. Two features that make HIV a more likely culprit than EBV, the most common cause of mononucleosis, are a morbilliform rash on the face and trunk in the absence of ampicillin therapy and oral ulcers. Preferred diagnostic tests are the HIV serology plus quantitative HIV RNA PCR (viral load) (45).

26. The most common infectious cause of **toxic megacolon** in patients with AIDS who are severely immunosuppressed is CMV infection (46).

27. Clinically, patients with AIDS with **PML** appear worse than their head magnetic resonance imaging (MRI) study, whereas the MRI in **HIV-associated dementia** appears worse than the patient (47,48).

28. Although **CMV pneumonitis** is a serious cause of morbidity and mortality in immunosuppressed bone marrow transplant patients, it is less clear whether it is a cause of clinically important pneumonia in patients

infected with HIV. The diagnosis of CMV pneumonitis requires that two conditions be met: (a) CMV is the sole pathogen recovered from bronchoalveolar lavage and transbronchial biopsy (i.e., no evidence of PCP infection) and (b) CMV nuclear inclusions (cytopathic effect) are seen on the transbronchial biopsy. A positive CMV culture from the bronchoalveolar lavage fluid indicates colonization, but is not diagnostic of CMV pneumonitis (49).

REFERENCES

1. Benhamou Y, Caumes E, Gerosa Y, et al. AIDS-related cholangiopathy. Critical analysis of a prospective series of 26 patients. *Dig Dis Sci* 1993;38:1113–1118.
2. Cello, JP. AIDS-related biliary tract disease. *Gastroint Endosc Clin N Am* 1998;8:963.
3. Cooper NB, Kenny W. Pulmonary complications in AIDS: the radiographic manifestations. *J Med Assoc Ga* 1989;78:197–200.
4. Anders HJ, Goebel FD. Cytomegalovirus polyradiculopathy in patients with AIDS. *Clin Infect Dis* 1998;27:345–352.
5. Armstrong WS, Katz JT, Kazanjian PH. Human immunodeficiency virus-associated fever of unknown origin: a study of 70 patients in the United States and review. *Clin Infect Dis* 1999;28:341–345.
6. Standiford KN, Emery CD, Schiffman RJ. Case report 865. Bacillary angiomatosis. *Skeletal Radiol* 1994;23:569–571.
7. Antinori A, Ammassari A, De Luca A, et al. Diagnosis of AIDS-related focal brain lesions: a decision-making analysis based on clinical and neuroradiologic characteristics combined with polymerase chain reaction assays in CSF. *Neurology* 1997;48:687–694.
8. Pierce MA, Johnson MD, Maciunas RJ, et al. Evaluating contrast-enhancing brain lesions in patients with AIDS by using positron emission tomography. *Ann Intern Med* 1995;123:594–598.
9. Carrazana EJ, Rossitch E Jr, Samuels MA. Cerebral toxoplasmosis In the acquired immune deficiency syndrome. *Clin Neurol Neurosurg* 1989;91:291–301.
10. Koduri PR, Kumapley R, Valladares J, et al. Chronic pure red cell aplasia caused by parvovirus B19 in AIDS: use of intravenous immunoglobulin–a report of eight patients. *Am J Hematol* 1999;61:16–20.

11. Case records of the Massachusetts General Hospital. Weekly clinicopathological exercises. Case 36—1993. A 28-year-old man with AIDS, persistent pancytopenia, and lymphoma. *N Engl J Med* 1993;329:792–799.

12. Kovacs JA, Ng VL, Masur H, et al. Diagnosis of *Pneumocystis carinii* pneumonia: improved detection in sputum with use of monoclonal antibodies. *N Engl J Med* 1988;318:589–593.

13. Salzman SH. Bronchoscopic techniques for the diagnosis of pulmonary complications of HIV infection. *Semin Respir Infect* 1999;14:318–326.

14. Cohen AH, Cohen GM. Distinguished Scientists Lecture Series. HIV-associated nephropathy. *Nephron* 1999;83:111–116.

15. Stone HD, Appel RG. Human immunodeficiency virus-associated nephropathy: current concepts. *Am J Med Sci* 1994;307:212–217.

16. Cunningham EE, Brentjens JR, Zielezny MA, et al. Heroin nephropathy. A clinicopathologic and epidemiologic study. *Am J Med* 1980;68:47–53.

17. Carbone L, D'Agati V, Cheng JT, et al. Course and prognosis of human immunodeficiency virus-associated nephropathy. *Am J Med* 1989;87:389–395.

18. Baker DJ, Reboli AC. Images in clinical medicine. Cutaneous cryptococcosis. *N Engl J Med* 1997;336:998.

19. Guardia JA, Ortiz-Butcher C, Bourgoignie JJ. Oncotic pressure and edema formation in hypoalbuminemic HIV-infected patients with proteinuria. *Am J Kidney Dis* 1997;30:822–828.

20. Williams DI, Williams DJ, Williams IG, et al. Presentation, pathology, and outcome of HIV associated renal disease in a specialist centre for HIV/AIDS. *Sex Transm Infect* 1998;74:179–184.

21. Ng VL, Yajko DM, Hadley WK. Extrapulmonary pneumocystosis. *Clin Microbiol Rev* 1997;10:401–418.

22. Ewig S, Schafer H, Rockstroh JK, et al. Effect of long-term primary aerosolized pentamidine prophylaxis on breakthrough *Pneumocystis carinii* pneumonia. *Eur Respir J* 1996;9:1006–1012.

23. Quist J, Hill AR. Serum lactate dehydrogenase (LDH) in *Pneumocystis carinii* pneumonia, tuberculosis, and bacterial pneumonia. *Chest* 1995;108:415–418.

24. Trachiotis GD, Vricella LA, Alyono D, et al. Management of AIDS-related pneumothorax [see comments]. *Ann Thorac Surg* 1996;62:1608–1613.

25. Steinman M, Steinman E, Poggetti RS, et al. Abdominal surgical emergencies in patients with acquired immunodeficiency syndrome. *Rev Assoc Med Bras* 1996;42:19–24.

26. Benson CA. Disease due to the *Mycobacterium avium* complex in patients with AIDS: epidemiology and clinical syndrome. *Clin Infect Dis* 1994;18[Suppl.3]:S218–S222.

27. Horsburgh CR Jr. *Mycobacterium avium* complex infection in the acquired immunodeficiency syndrome. *N Engl J Med* 1991; 324:1332–1338.

28. Fredricks DN, Rojanasthien N, Jacobson MA. AIDS-related disseminated histoplasmosis in San Francisco, California. *West J Med* 1997;167:315–321.

29. Wheat J. Histoplasmosis. Experience during outbreaks in Indianapolis and review of the literature. *Medicine* (Baltimore) 1997;76:339–354.

30. Wheat LJ, Kohler RB, Tewari RP. Diagnosis of disseminated histoplasmosis by detection of *Histoplasma capsulatum* antigen in serum and urine specimens. *N Engl J Med* 1986; 314:83–88.

31. Lai YP, Wu MS, Chen MY, et al. Timing and necessity of endoscopy in AIDS patients with dysphagia or odynophagia. *Hepatogastroenterology* 1998;45:2186–2189.

32. Wilcox CM. Esophageal disease in the acquired immunodeficiency syndrome: etiology, diagnosis, and management [see comments]. *Am J Med* 1992;92:412–421.

33. Moyle GJ, Sadler M. Peripheral neuropathy with nucleoside antiretrovirals: risk factors, incidence and management. *Drug Saf* 1998;19:481–494.

34. Graybill JR, Sobel J, Saag M, et al. Diagnosis and management of increased intracranial pressure in patients with AIDS and cryptococcal meningitis. The NIAID Mycoses Study Group and AIDS Cooperative Treatment Groups. *Clin Infect Dis* 2000;30:47–54.

35. Powderly WG. Cryptococcal meningitis and AIDS. *Clin Infect Dis* 1993;17:837–842.

36. Wang CY, Snow JL, Su WP. Lymphoma associated with human immunodeficiency virus infection [see comments]. *Mayo Clin Proc* 1995;70:665–672.

37. Bazot M, Cadranel J, Benayoun S, et al. Primary pulmonary AIDS-related lymphoma: radiographic and CT findings. *Chest* 1999;116:1282–1286.

38. Anders HJ, Goebel FD. Neurological manifestations of cytomegalovirus infection in the acquired immunodeficiency syndrome. *Int J STD AIDS* 1999;10:151–159.

39. Miller RF, Fox JD, Thomas P, et al. Acute lumbosacral polyradiculopathy due to cytomegalovirus in advanced HIV disease: CSF findings in 17 patients. *J Neurol Neurosurg Psychiatry* 1996;61:456–460.

40. Flegg PJ, Laing RB, Lee C, et al. Disseminated disease due to *Mycobacterium avium* complex in AIDS. *QJM* 1995;88: 617–626.

41. Nyberg DA, Federle MP, Jeffrey RB, et al. Abdominal CT findings of disseminated *Mycobacterium avium-intracellulare* in AIDS. *AJR Am J Roentgenol* 1985;145:297–299.

42. Chariot P, Drogou I, de Lacroix-Szmania I, et al. Zidovudine-induced mitochondrial disorder with massive liver steatosis, myopathy, lactic acidosis, and mitochondrial DNA depletion [see comments]. *J Hepatol* 1999;30:156–160.

43. Lenzo NP, Garas BA, French MA. Hepatic steatosis and lactic acidosis associated with stavudine treatment in an HIV patient: a case report [Letter]. *AIDS* 1997;11:1294–1296.

44. Fortgang IS, Belitsos PC, Chaisson RE, et al. Hepatomegaly and steatosis in HIV-infected patients receiving nucleoside analog antiretroviral therapy. *Am J Gastroenterol* 1995;90: 1433–1436.

45. Kahn JO, Walker BD. Acute human immunodeficiency virus type 1 infection. *N Engl J Med* 1998;339:33–39.

46. Davidson T, Allen-Mersh TG, Miles AJ, et al. Emergency laparotomy in patients with AIDS [see comments]. *Br J Surg* 1991;78:924–926.

47. Krupp LB, Lipton RB, Swerdlow ML, et al. Progressive multifocal leukoencephalopathy: clinical and radiographic features. *Ann Neurol* 1985;17:344–349.

48. Berger JR, Pall L, Lanska D, et al. Progressive multifocal leukoencephalopathy in patients with HIV infection. *J Neurovirol* 1998;4:59–68.

49. Salomon N, Perlman DC. Cytomegalovirus pneumonia. *Semin Respir Infect* 1999;14:353–358.

2

CARDIOLOGY

1. A regular, narrow complex tachycardia at 150 beats per minute (bpm) should suggest the possibility of **atrial flutter**. A saw-tooth pattern to the flutter waves, negative deflection in the inferior leads, and a regular flutter rate between 250 and 350 bpm support this diagnosis (1,2).

2. **Thrombolytics** do not decrease mortality in patients with a Killip IV myocardial infarction (MI; cardiogenic shock) (3).

3. **Thrombolytics** improve survival in patients who have an acute MI with electrocardiogram (ECG) changes demonstrating an ST-segment elevation >1 mm in two or more consecutive leads or a new left bundle branch block, provided the chest pain has not lasted >12 hours, absence of cardiogenic shock, and the patient has no absolute contraindications to thrombolytics (4).

4. **Polymorphic ventricular tachycardia (VT)** is an unstable rhythm and represents ischemia until proved otherwise (5–7).

5. The most important question to ask a patient with a **wide complex tachycardia** to distinguish VT from supraventricular tachycardia with aberrancy is whether the patient has a history of MI. If the answer is yes, there is a 95% chance that the arrhythmia is VT (8).

6. Although **flecainide** and other class I antiarrhythmics have been shown to increase mortality if given to patients with structural heart disease and arrhythmias, flecainide is a useful form of chemical cardioversion in patients with atrial fibrillation who otherwise have structurally normal hearts (9–11).

7. **Dressler syndrome** or postcardiac injury syndrome can manifest as fever, leukocytosis, pleuropericardial effusions, pericardial friction rub, and even pulmonary infiltrates. These features can occur from 1 week to months after an MI. Dressler syndrome is not limited to MI, but can also develop in patients with a recent history of chest surgery or pulmonary embolism (12).

8. A patient who presents with symptoms of MI who becomes hypotensive in response to a sublingual nitroglycerin may have a **right ventricular infarction** and be preload dependent. Inspect the inferior leads for ST-segment elevation, place right precordial leads to look for ST-segment elevation in lead RV_3 or RV_4, and be prepared to aggressively fluid resuscitate these patients (13,14).

9. Drugs that have shown a survival advantage in patients with an **acute ST-segment elevation MI** include aspirin, fibrinolytic agents, beta-blockers, and angiotensin converting enzyme (ACE) inhibitors (4).

10. Patients with **cardiac amyloidosis** should not be given digoxin or nifedipine. The amyloid fibrils, which bind digoxin, can lead to increased digoxin toxicity; nifedipine (as well as other after-load reducing agents) has led to hemodynamic compromise when given to patients with cardiac amyloid (15,16).

11. **Orthodeoxia** is a finding of arterial desaturation on standing. This is seen in a variety of diseases including right to left intracardiac shunt, pulmonary arteriovenous (AV) malformations seen with or without Osler-Weber-Rendu syndrome, cirrhosis, and recurrent pulmonary emboli (17–20).

12. Medications showing a survival benefit in patients with **congestive heart failure** (systolic dysfunction) include ACE inhibitors, isosorbide dinitrate in combination with hydralazine, β-blockers, and recently spironolactone (21–25).

13. A patient who presents with complaints of lower extremity claudication but has intact distal pulses may have **spinal stenosis**. One helpful clue is to attempt to

reproduce the pain by asking the patient to exercise. While the patient is exercising, feel for distal extremity pulses. The presence of intact pulses weighs heavily against claudication from arterial insufficiency (26).

14. **Atrioventricular nodal reentrant tachycardia** should be considered in a patient who presents with the abrupt onset of a regular, narrow complex tachycardia and prominent jugular venous a-waves that match the heart rate, a reflection of atrial contraction against a closed AV valve (27,28).

15. A patient with a history of **chronic atrial fibrillation** on digoxin who presents with a regular rhythm on ECG may have spontaneously converted to sinus rhythm or may be in a junctional rhythm from digoxin toxicity, leading to regularization of the R-R intervals (29,30).

16. Older men with symptoms of benign prostatic hypertrophy and symptomatic cardiac arrhythmias should avoid the **class I anti-arrhythmic disopyramide** because it has inherent anticholinergic properties that can lead to worsening urinary retention (31).

17. ST-segment depressions on ECG in the setting of **exercise treadmill testing (ETT)** are not predictive of coronary stenosis location. However, ST-segment elevations without Q waves, on ETT, are suggestive of coronary artery disease location (32–35).

18. **Hyperkalemia** is the most common metabolic cause of peaked T waves on 12-lead ECG. Peaked T waves may also be one of the earliest signs of acute cardiac ischemia (36).

19. If the outstretched arm length is greater than the patient's height, suspect **Marfan syndrome**. Other stigmata include high arched palate, pectus carinatum, ectopia lens, mitral valve prolapse, aortic regurgitation, thoracic aortic dissection, and family history (37–39).

20. The diastolic decrescendo murmur from **acute aortic dissection** or aneurysm is classically heard along the right sternal border, as opposed to **primary valvular aortic insufficiency** that can be heard best along the left sternal border (40,41).

21. Any patient on chronic amiodarone therapy who develops new atrial fibrillation, weight loss, worsening heart failure, or angina should be tested for **amiodarone-induced hyperthyroidism**. It is important to note that the atrial fibrillation can present with a normal ventricular rate, secondary to the intrinsic beta-blockade of amiodarone therapy (42).

22. In a patient with an **acute MI** who presents with ST-segment elevation, the ST-segment elevation is usually convex appearing and the T waves will classically invert before ST-segment normalization. In **acute pericarditis**, the ST-segment elevation normally appears concave, concomitant PR depression may be present, and the ST segments will normalize before T-wave inversion (43,44).

23. Patients with idiopathic **nonsustained VT** and no evidence of structural heart disease (normal ejection fraction) generally have an excellent prognosis, extremely low risk of sudden cardiac death, and do not typically benefit from automatic defibrillator placement (45,46).

24. In the presence of **digoxin toxicity**, electrolyte abnormalities, in particular hypokalemia, hypomagnesemia, and hypercalcemia, will exacerbate the systemic manifestations and dysrhythmias and should be corrected promptly (29,30).

25. An irregular wide complex tachycardia at rate >200 bpm should suggest atrial fibrillation with a rapid ventricular response down an accessory pathway. **Wolff-Parkinson-White syndrome** may be the underlying disease process. Avoid AV nodal blocking agents (e.g., digoxin or calcium channel blockers) which can speed up the conduction through the accessory pathway (47).

26. The most common ECG abnormality in **arrhythmogenic right ventricular dysplasia** is T-wave inversions in the precordial leads. This diagnosis should be entertained in any patient without coronary heart disease who presents in monomorphic sustained on

non-sustained VT or in patients who present with exertional syncope. One helpful imaging tool is a magnetic resonance imaging study, which shows a paper-thin right ventricular free wall and fatty replacement of the right ventricular myocardium. This is an important diagnosis to make because an automatic implantable cardioverter-defibrillator (AICD) placement in these patients may saves lives (48–52).

27. Some features that help distinguish **cardiac tamponade** from **constrictive pericarditis** are the presence of hypotension, distant heart sounds, pulsus paradoxus, electrical alternans on ECG, pericardial effusion, and right atrial and right ventricular diastolic collapse on echocardiography, which all favor cardiac tamponade. Kussmaul sign, pericardial knock, thickened pericardium on echocardiogram, and pericardial calcification favor constrictive pericarditis. Note that equalization of cardiac chamber pressures is usually seen in both disorders (53–55).

28. An inverted P wave in lead V_1, a large R wave in V_1, and deep S waves in V_5 and V_6 in a patient with chronic dyspnea and intermittent hemoptysis should raise suspicion for **mitral stenosis** (56).

29. **AV dissociation** in a regular wide complex tachycardia can help point to VT as the cause of the rhythm abnormality (57).

30. Consider the diagnosis of **peripartum cardiomyopathy** in a woman who presents with signs and symptoms of heart failure after 36 weeks of gestation up to 5 months postpartum. It should be noted that patients with preexisting ischemic, valvular, or myopathic cardiac disease typically manifest cardiac disease during the second trimester, which is the period in pregnancy that places the greatest hemodynamic stress on the heart. On echocardiography, the overall ejection fraction is compromised in peripartum cardiomyopathy (58).

31. The differential diagnosis of **low voltage** on an ECG consists of those entities that place distance between

the leads and the myocardium: air (pneumothorax and chronic obstructive pulmonary disease), water (pericardial effusion), blood (cardiac tamponade), infiltrative diseases (amyloid, sarcoid, hemochromatosis), fat (obesity), as well as hypothyroidism and coronary artery disease (59).

32. An R wave in lead V_1 and V_2 with associated ST-segment flattening or depressions and upright T waves in a patient with chest pain should heighten suspicion for a **posterior MI**. The posterior infarction is most commonly associated with ST-segment elevations in the inferior leads (60,61).

33. A patient who on ECG demonstrates right bundle branch block (RBBB) with chronic ST-segment elevation in leads V_1–V_3 may be at risk for ventricular fibrillation and sudden cardiac death. This condition is referred to as **Brugada syndrome**. These patients do benefit from an AICD (62,63).

34. Consider the diagnosis of **right ventricular infarction** if the patient presents with the triad of CP, JVD, and a clear chest x-ray study (13,14).

35. **Digibind** is recommended for patients with super-therapeutic digoxin levels and symptomatic tachy- or bradyarrhythmias. Be aware of the patient with worsening renal failure who was given Digibind, because as both Digibind and digoxin are cleared renally an initial improvement may be seen with subsequent rebound bradycardia (29,30).

36. **ST-segment depressions** do not have localizing value with regard to coronary distribution (34,35).

37. The differential diagnosis of a **dominant R wave** in V_1 is a posterior MI, right ventricular hypertrophy, RBBB, Duchenne muscular dystrophy, Wolff-Parkinson-White syndrome, dextrocardia, and normal variant (64).

38. Following MI in a patient with an interpretable ECG, the absence of prior Q waves, AWMI as the index MI, prior congestive heart failure or congestive heart failure in the critical care unit predicts an **ejection fraction >40%** with high predictive value (65).

REFERENCES

1. Waldo AL. Treatment of atrial flutter. *Heart* 2000;84:227–232.
2. Daoud EG, Morady F. Pathophysiology of atrial flutter. *Annu. Rev.Med.* 1998;49:77–83.
3. Lee KL, Woodlief LH, Topol EJ, et al. Predictors of 30-day mortality in the era of reperfusion for acute myocardial infarction. Results from an international trial of 41,021 patients. GUSTO-I Investigators [see comments]. *Circulation* 1995;91: 1659–1668.
4. Ryan TJ, Anderson JL, Antman EM, et al. ACC/AHA guidelines for the management of patients with acute myocardial infarction. A report of the American College of Cardiology/ American Heart Association Task Force on Practice Guidelines (Committee on Management of Acute Myocardial Infarction). *J Am Coll Cardiol* 1996;28:1328–1428.
5. Stern EH, Schweitzer P. Polymorphous ventricular tachycardia associated with acute myocardial infarction [Letter, comment]. *Circulation* 1992;85:2333–2334.
6. Wolfe CL, Nibley C, Bhandari A, et al. Polymorphous ventricular tachycardia associated with acute myocardial infarction [see comments]. *Circulation* 1991;84:1543–1551.
7. Eldar M, Sievner Z, Goldbourt U, et al. Primary ventricular tachycardia in acute myocardial infarction: clinical characteristics and mortality. The SPRINT Study Group [see comments]. *Ann Intern Med* 1992;117:31–36.
8. Shah CP, Thakur RK, Xie B, et al. Clinical approach to wide QRS complex tachycardias. *Emerg Med Clin North Am* 1998; 16:331–360.
9. The Cardiac Arrhythmia Suppression Trial (CAST) Investigators. Preliminary report: effect of encainide and flecainide on mortality in a randomized trial of arrhythmia suppression after myocardial infarction [see comments]. *N Engl J Med* 1989; 321:406–412.
10. Echt DS, Liebson PR, Mitchell LB, et al Mortality and morbidity in patients receiving encainide, flecainide, or placebo. The Cardiac Arrhythmia Suppression Trial [see comments]. *N Engl J Med* 1991;324:781–788.
11. Falk RH, Fogel RI. Flecainide. *J Cardiovasc Electrophysiol* 1994;5:964–981.
12. Dressler W. The post-myocardial infarction syndrome. *Arch Intern Med* 1994;103:28–42.

13. Goldstein JA. Right heart ischemia: pathophysiology, natural history, and clinical management. *Prog Cardiovasc Dis* 1998; 40:325–341.

14. Goldstein JA. Pathophysiology and clinical management of right heart ischemia. *Curr Opin Cardiol* 1999;14:329–339.

15. Gertz MA, Skinner M, Connors LH, et al Selective binding of nifedipine to amyloid fibrils. *Am J Cardiol* 1985;55:1646.

16. Rubinow A, Skinner M, Cohen AS. Digoxin sensitivity in amyloid cardiomyopathy. *Circulation* 1981;63:1285–1288.

17. Faller M, Kessler R, Chaouat A, et al. Platypnea-orthodeoxia syndrome related to an aortic aneurysm combined with an aneurysm of the atrial septum. *Chest* 2000;118:553–557.

18. Kubler P, Gibbs H, Garrahy P. Platypnoea-orthodeoxia syndrome. *Heart* 2000;83:221–223.

19. Lambrecht GL, Malbrain ML, Coremans P, et al. Orthodeoxia and platypnea in liver cirrhosis: effects of propranolol. *Acta Clin Belg* 1994;49:26–30.

20. Cheng TO. Reversible orthodeoxia [Letter, comment]. *Ann Intern Med* 1992;116:875.

21. Pitt B, Zannad F, Remme WJ, et al. The effect of spironolactone on morbidity and mortality in patients with severe heart failure. Randomized Aldactone Evaluation Study Investigators [see comments]. *N Engl J Med* 1999;341:709–717.

22. Frantz RP. Beta blockade in patients with congestive heart failure. Why, who, and how. *Postgrad Med* 2000;108: 103–110, 116.

23. Elkayam U. Nitrates in the treatment of congestive heart failure. *Am J Cardiol* 1996;77:41C–51C.

24. Cohn JN. Nitrates versus angiotensin-converting enzyme inhibitors for congestive heart failure. *Am J Cardiol* 1993;72: 21C–24C.

25. Cohn JN. Heart failure: future treatment approaches. *Am J Hypertens* 2000;13:74S–78S.

26. Porter RW. Spinal stenosis and neurogenic claudication. *Spine* 1996;21:2046–2052.

27. Karas BJ, Grubb BP. Reentrant tachycardias. A look at where treatment stands today. *Postgrad Med* 1998;103:84–86, 98.

28. Elvas L, Gursoy S, Brugada J, et al. Atrioventricular nodal reentrant tachycardia: a review. *Can J Cardiol* 1994;10:342–348.

29. Kelly RA, Smith TW. Recognition and management of digitalis toxicity. *Am J Cardiol* 1992;69:108G–118G.

30. Taboulet P, Baud FJ, Bismuth C. Clinical features and management of digitalis poisoning—rationale for immuno-therapy [see comments]. *J Toxicol Clin Toxicol* 1993;31: 247–260.

31. Alves LE, Rose EP, Cahill TB Jr, et al. Disopyramide-induced urinary retention [Letter]. *Arch Intern Med* 1984;144:2099.

32. Kurata C, Tawarahara K, Okayama K, et al. Localization of exercise-induced myocardial ischemia with ST depression. *Intern Med* 1992;31:583–588.

33. Gallik DM, Mahmarian JJ, Verani MS. Therapeutic significance of exercise-induced ST-segment elevation in patients without previous myocardial infarction [see comments]. *Am J Cardiol* 1993;72:1–7.

34. Longhurst JC, Kraus WL. Exercise-induced ST elevation in patients without myocardial infarction. *Circulation* 1979;60:616–629.

35. Kang X, Berman DS, Lewin HC, et al. Comparative localization of myocardial ischemia by exercise electrocardiography and myocardial perfusion SPECT. *J Nucl Cardiol* 2000;7:140–145.

36. Kuvin JT. Images in clinical medicine. Electrocardiographic changes of hyperkalemia. *N Engl J Med* 1998;338:662.

37. Pyeritz RE. The Marfan syndrome. *Annu Rev Med* 2000;51:481–510.

38. von Kodolitsch Y, Schwartz AG, Nienaber CA. Clinical prediction of acute aortic dissection. *Arch Intern Med* 2000;160:2977–2982.

39. Cooke JP, Safford RE. Progress in the diagnosis and management of aortic dissection. *Mayo Clin Proc* 1986;61:147–153.

40. Isselbacher E, Eagl K, Desanctis R. Diseases of the aorta. In: Braunwald E, ed. *Heart disease: a textbook of cardiovascular medicine.* Philadelphia: WB Saunders, 2000:1555–1569.

41. Slater EE, DeSanctis RW. The clinical recognition of dissecting aortic aneurysm. *Am J Med* 1976;60:625–633.

42. Harjai KJ, Licata AA. Effects of amiodarone on thyroid function [see comments]. *Ann Intern Med* 1997;126:63–73.

43. Baljepally R, Spodick DH. PR-segment deviation as the initial electrocardiographic response in acute pericarditis. *Am J Cardiol* 1998;81:1505–1506.

44. Marinella MA. Electrocardiographic manifestations and differential diagnosis of acute pericarditis. *Am Fam Physician* 1998;57:699–704.

45. Lerman BB, Stein KM, Markowitz SM, et al. Ventricular arrhythmias in normal hearts. *Cardiol Clin* 2000;18:265–291, vii.

46. Lerman BB, Stein KM, Markowitz SM. Idiopathic right ventricular outflow tract tachycardia: a clinical approach. *Pacing Clin Electrophysiol* 1996;19:2120–2137.

47. Moore GP, Munter DW. Wolff-Parkinson-White syndrome: illustrative case and brief review. *J Emerg Med* 1989;7:47–54.

48. Al Khatib SM, Pritchett EL. Clinical features of Wolff-Parkinson-White syndrome. *Am Heart J* 1999;138:403–413.

49. Cohen TJ, Zadeh H, Fruauff A, et al. Arrhythmogenic right ventricular dysplasia and the implantable cardioverter-defibrillator: a case report and review of the literature. *J Invasive Cardiol* 2000;12:422–424.

50. van der Wall EE, Kayser HW, Bootsma MM, et al. Arrhythmogenic right ventricular dysplasia: MRI findings. *Herz* (Muchen) 2000;25:356–364.

51. Corrado D, Basso C, Thiene G. Arrhythmogenic right ventricular cardiomyopathy: diagnosis, prognosis, and treatment. *Heart* 2000;83:588–595.

52. Corrado D, Fontaine G, Marcus FI, et al. Arrhythmogenic right ventricular dysplasia/cardiomyopathy: need for an international registry. Study Group on Arrhythmogenic Right Ventricular Dysplasia/Cardiomyopathy of the Working Groups on Myocardial and Pericardial Disease and Arrhythmias of the European Society of Cardiology and of the Scientific Council on Cardiomyopathies of the World Heart Federation. *Circulation* 2000;101:E101–E106.

53. Myers RB, Spodick DH. Constrictive pericarditis: clinical and pathophysiologic characteristics. *Am Heart J* 1999;138: 219–232.

54. Tsang TS, Oh JK, Seward JB. Diagnosis and management of cardiac tamponade in the era of echocardiography. *Clin Cardiol* 1999;22:446–452.

55. Brockington GM, Zebede J, Pandian NG. Constrictive pericarditis. *Cardiol Clin* 1990;8:645–661.

56. Braunwald E. Valvular heart disease. In: Braunwald E, ed. *Heart disease: a textbook of cardiovascular medicine.* Philadelphia: WB Saunders, 1997:1011–1012.

57. Wellens HJ, Bar FW, Lie KI. The value of the electrocardiogram in the differential diagnosis of a tachycardia with a widened QRS complex. *Am J Med* 1978;64:27–33.

58. Lampert MB, Lang RM. Peripartum cardiomyopathy [see comments]. *Am Heart J* 1995;130:860–870.

59. Sweetwood HM. The clinical significance of low QRS voltage. *Critical Care Nurse* 1997;17:73–78.

60. Brady WJ. Acute posterior wall myocardial infarction: electrocardiographic manifestations. *Am J Emerg Med* 1998;16: 409–413.

61. Casas RE, Marriott HJ, Glancy DL. Value of leads V7–V9 in diagnosing posterior wall acute myocardial infarction and other causes of tall R waves in V1–V2. *Am J Cardiol* 1997; 80:508–509.

62. Brugada P, Brugada R, Brugada J. The Brugada syndrome. *Curr Cardiol Rep* 2000;2:507–514.
63. Gussak I, Antzelevitch C, Bjerregaard P, et al. The Brugada syndrome: clinical, electrophysiologic and genetic aspects. *J Am Coll Cardiol* 1999;33:5–15.
64. Nikolic G. Dominant R wave in lead V1. *Heart Lung* 1998;27:352–353.
65. Peterson ED, Shaw LJ, Califf RM. Risk stratification after myocardial infarction [see comments]. *Ann Intern Med* 1997;126:561–582.

3

DERMATOLOGY

1. Up to 40% of patients who present with **erythema nodosum** (painful erythematous subcutaneous nodules on extensor surface of legs) will have no associated abnormality (1,2).

2. Rashes that affect the **palms and soles** are helpful because they generally limit the differential diagnosis to gonococcemia, Rocky Mountain spotted fever, erythema multiforme, and secondary syphilis (3,4).

3. The differential diagnosis of **erythroderma** is toxic shock syndrome, Sézary syndrome, exacerbation of preexisting psoriasis, seborrheic dermatitis, atopic dermatitis, pityriasis rubra pilaris, drug reaction, and paraneoplastic syndromes. Morbidity from erythroderma occurs from bacterial superinfection leading to sepsis, high output heart failure, and protein loss. Much erythroderma remains undefined (5,6).

4. **Livedo reticularis**, a netlike pattern of cyanosis that blanches with pressure, is rarely an isolated abnormality. It is also seen in conjunction with Raynaud's phenomenon, or may reflect systemic disease such as systemic lupus erythematosus (SLE), dermatomyositis, rheumatoid arthritis, polyarteritis nodosa, and, in particular, antiphospholipid antibody syndrome and cholesterol emboli syndrome (7).

5. Consider **Sneddon syndrome** in a patient with livedo reticularis and a history of multiple cerebral vascular accidents. The cause of this disease is unknown (8–11).

6. **Nailfold capillary dilation** should suggest three disease processes: dermatomyositis, scleroderma, and SLE. Of these, it is most prominent in dermatomyositis. Rheumatoid arthritis does not dilate the nailfold capillary (12,15).

7. **Scabies** is the most pruritic dermatologic rash. Classically, the itching is worse at night and after hot showers. Inspect the volar aspect of the wrists, between the fingers, elbows, and penis for small papules and vesicles. The face, scalp, neck, palms, and soles are generally spared except in infants. Bacterial superinfection with streptococci has led to acute poststreptococcal glomerulonephritis. Crusted or Norwegian scabies is a hyperinfestation with thousands to millions of mites that target immunodeficient patients. Crusted scabies may appear similar to psoriasis in its erythematous appearance with thick keratotic crusts. This form of scabies is highly contagious but difficult to diagnose because it is not always pruritic (16–18).

8. Think of herpes simplex virus as an underlying cause of **recurrent erythema multiforme minor** (target lesions with little mucosal involvement) (19,20).

9. **Pathergy** is the presence of an erythematous papule or pustule at least 5 mm in size that appears 24 to 48 hours after local skin trauma or a skin prick. It is one of the major criteria for the diagnosis of Behçet syndrome, but can also be seen in pyoderma gangrenosum (21,22).

10. In patients with redness and scaling of one palm, the next step is to examine both feet, which may show redness and scaling in a moccasin-type distribution. This distribution is characteristic of the **two feet-one hand syndrome** of *Trichophyton* fungal infection (bilateral *Tinea pedis* and unilateral *T. manuum*) (23–25).

11. The combination of buttock—lower extremity palpable purpura, abdominal pain, hematuria, renal insufficiency, and arthralgia or arthritis is suggestive of **Henoch-Schönlein purpura**. Definitive diagnosis can be made by biopsy of skin demonstrating IgA deposition by immunofluorescence and small vessel leuko-

cytoclastic vasculitis predominantly in postcapillary venules (26,27).

12. **Pityriasis rosea** is an erythematous scaling eruption that often begins with a larger herald patch followed by smaller pink oval scaling papules in a Christmas tree pattern. One systemic infection that can mimic pityriasis rosea is **secondary syphilis**, which can be ruled out by ordering a rapid plasma reagin (RPR) test. The presence of a herald patch makes pityriasis rosea the likely diagnosis (28,29).

13. Tuberous sclerosis, neurofibromatosis, von Hippel-Lindau syndrome, and Sturge-Weber syndrome represent **phakomatoses** that are neurocutaneous diseases. Tuberous sclerosis is characterized by the tetrad of mental retardation, seizures, adenoma sebaceum (papulonodules on the face), and ash-leaflet white spots (hypopigmented macules). Neurofibromatosis has two forms NF1 and NF2. Both are manifested by café-au-lait macules and neurofibromas; however, only NF1 has pigmented hamartomas of the iris (Lisch nodules) and bilateral acoustic neuromas are seen only in NF2. Retinal and cerebellar hemangioblastomas, renal cell carcinoma, and pheochromocytoma characterize Von Hippel-Lindau syndrome. Sturge-Weber syndrome is characterized by port-wine stain along the trigeminal distribution of the face and intracranial calcifications. Seizures are one of the feared complications of this disorder (30–36).

14. **Gottron papules** are violaceous, flat-topped papules typically found over the metacarpophalangeal, distal interphalangeal, and proximal interphalangeal joints of the hands of patients with dermatomyositis. Periungual telangiectasias invariably can be found in patients with Gottron papules and the absence of periungual telangiectasias precludes the diagnosis of dermatomyositis (37).

15. Multiple sebaceous adenomas on the head, neck, and trunk may be associated with internal malignancy, most commonly involving the colon. The eponym is **Muir-Torre syndrome** (38).

16. Supraorbital violaceous erythema with edema in a patient with proximal muscle weakness is highly suggestive of dermatomyositis. The periorbital erythema is referred to as the **heliotrope rash** and is virtually pathognomonic for dermatomyositis (37).

17. The only clinical clue to **necrotizing fasciitis** may be severe pain in an extremity out of proportion to cutaneous erythema. Necrotizing fasciitis is often accompanied by leukocytosis with bandemia and fever, although these findings can resemble cellulitis. The most common organism is group A streptococcus. Once violaceous bullae develop, the infection is far advanced (39–42).

18. Pruritic, bilateral, grouped papulovesicles on the extensor surfaces of the elbows and knees, as well as the buttocks, are a clue to the presence of **dermatitis herpetiformis**. Direct immunofluorescence adjacent to affected skin demonstrates IgA deposits along the basement membrane. Testing for IgA antiendomysial antibodies is also useful for diagnosis and prognosis of this condition. It is important to note that gluten-sensitive enteropathy is found in almost all cases of dermatitis herpetiformis (43).

19. **Acquired ichthyosis** is a fine, fish scalelike pattern of hyperkeratosis that can be a sign of systemic disease, including Hodgkin disease (most common malignancy), human immunodeficiency virus (HIV), sarcoidosis, SLE, dermatomyositis, as well as other malignancies (44–46).

20. Discovering perifollicular hemorrhages amidst corkscrew hair is the sine qua non of **scurvy** (47).

21. The presence of hypopigmented, anesthetic macules should raise suspicion for the chronic granulomatous disease, **leprosy**, caused by *Mycobacterium leprae* (48,49).

22. Infectious diseases associated with *erythema nodosum* include beta-hemolytic streptococcal pharyngitis, tuberculosis, leprosy, endemic fungi (e.g., coccidioidomycosis), Epstein-Barr virus, yersiniosis, bartonellosis, and brucellosis (50).

23. **Pemphigus vulgaris (PV)** is one of the autoimmune blistering diseases characterized by intraepidermal flaccid blisters on normal or erythematous appearing skin. The blisters rupture easily and pressure applied to the lateral margins of the blisters can cause the separation of the epidermis termed **Nikolsky sign**. Oral involvement with PV is the rule. PV can be life threatening. Before steroid therapy was available the mortality rate was between 60% to 90%. It is currently 5% to 15% (51).

24. **Bullous pemphigoid** is an autoimmune, subepidermal blistering disorder characterized by tense blisters in the elderly. Nikolsky sign is absent and, although glucocorticoids are first-line treatment, mortality rate is low even in the absence of therapy (51).

25. If a patient with straight hair and severe acne presents with **spontaneously curling hair**, it is most likely a side effect of isotretinoin therapy (52,53).

26. Consider the diagnosis of **Fabry disease** in a young adult male who presents with purplish-red papules in a bathing suit distribution associated with exquisite shooting pains in the lower extremities. The skin rash is termed "angiokeratoma corporis diffusum." Renal insufficiency may be present (54–56).

27. Consider the diagnosis of HIV in any patient who presents with **molluscum contagiosum** of the face. Molluscum contagiosum typically appears as skin-colored umbilicated papules. Consider disseminated cryptococcosis in an HIV-positive patient with a CD4 count less than 100 cells/mm³ who appears systemically ill with multiple skin lesions resembling molluscum (57–60).

28. If a patient presents with linear, erythematous subdermal and subcutaneous nodules on one extremity, ask about a recent history of gardening, in particular whether pricked by a rose thorn. The lymphangitis is caused by the fungus ***Sporothrix schenckii*** (61).

29. **Scarlet fever** can be more challenging to discern in black patients because of the less intense erythema.

It may be important to palpate the sandpaper quality of the rash and look for other findings, including white or red strawberry tongue, linear petechiae in the antecubital fossa known as "Pastia sign," palatal petechiae, desquamation of the involved skin, pharyngitis, and circumoral pallor (62).

30. Hyperglycemia in association with an inflammatory, scaly rash should lead to the diagnosis of **glucagonoma syndrome**. Necrolytic migratory erythema (NME) is the name of the rash that begins as erythematous papules or plaques on the face, extremities, and perineum. The lesions often coalesce with central clearing and characteristically have a scaling border. Hyperglycemia and NME are the two most common features of this unusual neuroendocrine tumor (63–65).

31. **Cutaneous T-cell lymphoma (CTCL)** should be considered in the differential diagnosis of patients who present with eczema or psoriasis refractory to treatment. An increase in the palpable component of the underlying plaque of "eczema" may serve as a clue to the presence of the CTCL (66–69).

32. In a patient with **cutaneous plaque psoriasis** and hypertension, treatment of the blood pressure with beta-blockers and angiotensin-converting enzyme inhibitors may result in exacerbation of the psoriasis (70–72).

33. A number of dermatologic conditions are associated with **hepatitis C virus**: cryoglobulinemic vasculitis, porphyria cutanea tarda, and lichen planus (73).

34. The most important prognostic factor regarding **cutaneous melanoma** is tumor thickness (74,75).

35. The two most common systemic diseases associated with chronic lower extremity **palpable purpura** are Henoch-Schönlein purpura in children and cryoglobulinemia in adults (76–79).

36. A sudden, increased number of seborrheic keratoses in a patient with gastrointestinal complaints (early satiety, abdominal pain, constipation, anemia, change in

stool caliber) suggests gastrointestinal malignancy. This is termed the sign of **Leser-Trelat**. It may be seen in association with numerous skin tags or acanthosis nigricans (80,81).

REFERENCES

1. Farraj R, Colville DS. 57-year old woman with anemia and rash. *Mayo Clin Proc* 1996;71:303–306.
2. Garcia-Porrua C, Gonzalez-Gay MA, Vazquez-Caruncho M, et al. Erythema nodosum: etiologic and predictive factors in a defined population. *Arthritis Rheum* 2000;43:584–592.
3. Schlossberg D. Fever and rash. *Infect Dis Clin North Am* 1996;10:101–110.
4. Salzman MB, Rubin LG. Meningococcemia. *Infect Dis Clin North Am* 1996;10:709–725.
5. Sigurdsson V, Toonstra J, Hezemans-Boer M, et al. Erythroderma: a clinical and follow-up study of 102 patients, with special emphasis on survival. *J Am Acad Dermatol* 1996;35:53–57.
6. Sigurdsson V, Toonstra J, van Vloten WA. Idiopathic erythroderma: a follow-up study of 28 patients. *Dermatology* 1997;194:98–101.
7. Gibson GE, Su WP, Pittelkow MR. Antiphospholipid syndrome and the skin. *J Am Acad Dermatol* 1997;36:970–982.
8. Frances CT, Papo B, Wechsler JL, et al. Sneddon syndrome with or without antiphospholipid antibodies. A comparative study in 46 patients. *Medicine (Baltimore)* 1999;78:209–219.
9. Yell JA, Mbuagbaw J, Burge SM. Cutaneous manifestations of systemic lupus erythematosus. *Br J Dermatol* 1996;135:355–362.
10. Sabatine MS, Oelberg DA, Mark EJ, et al. Pulmonary cholesterol crystal embolization. *Chest* 1997;112:1687–1692.
11. Gibson LE, Su WP. Cutaneous vasculitis. *Rheum Dis Clin North Am* 1995;21:1097–1113.
12. ter Borg EJ, Piersma-Wichers G, Smit AJ, et al. Serial nailfold capillary microscopy in primary Raynaud's phenomenon and scleroderma. *Semin Arthritis Rheum* 1994;24:40–47.
13. Ganczarczyk ML, Lee P, Armstrong SK. Nailfold capillary microscopy in polymyositis and dermatomyositis. *Arthritis Rheum* 1988;31:116–119.
14. Kabasakal Y, Elvins DM, Ring EF, et al. Quantitative nailfold capillaroscopy findings in a population with connective tissue disease and in normal healthy controls. *Ann Rheum Dis* 1996;55:507–512.

15. Lee P, Leung FY, Alderdice C, et al. Nailfold capillary microscopy in the connective tissue diseases: a semiquantitative assessment. *J Rheumatol* 1983;10:930–938.
16. Rosen T, Brown TJ. Cutaneous manifestations of sexually transmitted diseases. *Med Clin North Am* 1998;82:1081–1104, vi.
17. Schlesinger I, Oelrich DM, Tyring SK. Crusted (Norwegian) scabies in patients with AIDS: the range of clinical presentations. *South Med J* 1994;87:352–356.
18. Reid HF, Birju B, Holder Y, et al. Epidemic scabies in four Caribbean islands, 1981–1988. *Trans R Soc Trop Med Hyg* 1990;84:298–300.
19. Schofield JK, Tatnall FM, Brown J, et al. Recurrent erythema multiforme: tissue typing in a large series of patients. *Br J Dermatol* 1994;131:532–535.
20. Schofield JK, Tatnall FM, Leigh IM. Recurrent erythema multiforme: clinical features and treatment in a large series of patients. *Br J Dermatol* 1993;128:542–545.
21. Krause I, Molad Y, Mitrani M, et al. Pathergy reaction in Behçet's disease: lack of correlation with mucocutaneous manifestations and systemic disease expression. *Clin Exp Rheumatol* 2000;18:71–74.
22. Akmaz O, Erel A, Gurer MA. Comparison of histopathologic and clinical evaluations of pathergy test in Behçet's disease. *Int J Dermatol* 2000;39:121–125.
23. Singri P, Brodell RT. 'Two feet-one hand' syndrome. A recurring infection with a peculiar connection. *Postgrad Med* 1999;106:83–84.
24. Seeburger J, Scher RK. Long-term remission of two feet-one hand syndrome. *Cutis* 1998;61:149–151.
25. Daniel CR III, Gupta AK, Daniel MP, et al. Two feet-one hand syndrome: a retrospective multicenter survey. *Int J Dermatol* 1997;36:658–660.
26. Saulsbury FT. Henoch-Schönlein purpura in children. Report of 100 patients and review of the literature. *Medicine (Baltimore)* 1999;78:395–409.
27. Blanco R, Martinez-Taboada VM, Rodriguez-Valverde V, et al. Henoch-Schönlein purpura in adulthood and childhood: two different expressions of the same syndrome [see comments]. *Arthritis Rheum* 1997;40:859–864.
28. Secher L, Weismann K, Kobayasi T. Pityriasis rosea eruption in secondary syphilis: an isomorphic phenomenon? *Cutis* 1985;35:403–404.
29. Stillman MA. Papulosquamous diseases. *Prim Care* 1978;5:197–213.
30. Case records of the Massachusetts General Hospital. Weekly clinicopathological exercises. Case 18-1994. A 37-year-old

woman with interstitial lung disease, renal masses, and a previous spontaneous pneumothorax [clinical conference] [see comments] [published erratum appears in *N Engl J Med* 1995; 332(21):1455]. *N Engl J Med* 1994;330:1300–1306.

31. Roach ES, DiMario FJ, Kandt RS, et al. Tuberous Sclerosis Consensus Conference: recommendations for diagnostic evaluation. National Tuberous Sclerosis Association. *J Child Neurol* 1999;14:401–407.

32. Roach ES, Gomez MR, Northrup H. Tuberous sclerosis complex consensus conference: revised clinical diagnostic criteria. *J Child Neurol* 1998;13:624–628.

33. Hurst JS, Wilcoski S. Recognizing an index case of tuberous sclerosis. *Am Fam Physician* 2000;61:703–708, 710.

34. Gutmann DH, Aylsworth A, Carey JC, et al. The diagnostic evaluation and multidisciplinary management of neurofibromatosis 1 and neurofibromatosis 2 [see comments]. *JAMA* 1997;278:51–57.

35. Maher ER, Kaelin WG Jr. von Hippel-Lindau disease. *Medicine (Baltimore)* 1997;76:381–391.

36. Mirowski GW, Liu AA, Stone ML, et al. Sturge-Weber syndrome. *J Am Acad Dermatol* 1999;41:772–773.

37. Callen JP. Dermatomyositis. *Lancet* 2000;355:53–57.

38. Ward SK, Roenigk HH, Gordon KB. Dermatologic manifestations of gastrointestinal disorders. *Gastroenterol Clin North Am* 1998;27:615–636, vi.

39. Meltzer DL, Kabongo M. Necrotizing fasciitis: a diagnostic challenge. *Am Fam Physician* 1997;56:145–149.

40. Stone DR, Gorbach. SL. Necrotizing fasciitis. The changing spectrum. *Dermatol Clin* 1997;15:213–220.

41. Green RJ, Dafoe DC, Raffin TA. Necrotizing fasciitis. *Chest* 1996;110:219–229.

42. Kotrappa KS, Bansal RS, Amin NM. Necrotizing fasciitis [published erratum appears in *Am Fam Physician* 1997;55(2):448]. *Am Fam Physician* 1996;53:1691–1697.

43. Reunala T. Dermatitis herpetiformis: coeliac disease of the skin [Editorial]. *Ann Med* 1998;30:416–418.

44. Brenner S. Acquired ichthyosis in AIDS. *Cutis* 1987;39:421–423.

45. Urrutia S, Vazquez F, Requena L, et al. Acquired ichthyosis associated with dermatomyositis [Letter]. *J Am Acad Dermatol* 1987;16:627–629.

46. Schwartz RA, Williams ML. Acquired ichthyosis: a marker for internal disease. *Am Fam Physician* 1984;29:181–184.

47. Hirschmann JV, Raugi GJ. Adult scurvy. *J Am Acad Dermatol* 1999;41:895–906.

48. Case records of the Massachusetts General Hospital. Weekly clinicopathological exercises. Case 49-1985. A 25-year-old

Haitian man with Hansen's disease, painful subcutaneous nodules, fever, and hypesthesia. *N Engl J Med* 1985;313: 1464–1472.

49. Jacobson RR, Krahenbuhl JL. Leprosy. Lancet 1999;353: 655–660.

50. Cribier B, Caille A, Heid E, et al. Erythema nodosum and associated diseases. A study of 129 cases. *Int J Dermatol* 1998;37:667–672.

51. Scott JE, Ahmed AR. The blistering diseases. *Med Clin North Am* 1998;82:1239–1283.

52. van der Pijl JW, Bavinck JN, de Fijter JW. Isotretinoin and azathioprine: a synergy that makes hair curl? [Letter]. *Lancet* 1996;348:622–623.

53. Bunker CB, Maurice PD, Dowd PM. Isotretinoin and curly hair. *Clin Exp Dermatol* 1990;15:143–145.

54. Case 2-1984: Fabry's disease [Letter]. *N Engl J Med* 1984; 310:1607.

55. Kato H, Sato K, Hattori S, et al. Fabry's disease. *Intern Med* 1992;31:682–685.

56. Peters FP, Sommer A, Vermeulen A, et al. Fabry's disease: a multidisciplinary disorder. *Postgrad Med J* 1997;73:710–712.

57. Ficarra G, Cortes S, Rubino I, et al. Facial and perioral molluscum contagiosum in patients with HIV infection. A report of eight cases. *Oral Surg Oral Med Oral Pathol* 1994;78: 621–626.

58. Munoz-Perez MA, Colmenero MA, Rodriguez-Pichardo A, et al. Disseminated cryptococcosis presenting as molluscum-like lesions as the first manifestation of AIDS. *Int J Dermatol* 1996; 35:646–648.

59. Murakawa GJ, Kerschmann R, Berger T. Cutaneous cryptococcus infection and AIDS. Report of 12 cases and review of the literature. *Arch Dermatol* 1996;132:545–548.

60. Chiewchanvit S, Chuaychoo B, Mahanupab P. Disseminated cryptococcosis presenting as molluscum-like lesions in three male patients with acquired immunodeficiency syndrome. *J Med Assoc Thai* 1994;77:322–326.

61. Davis BA. Sporotrichosis. *Dermatol Clin* 1996;14:69–76.

62. Manders SM. Toxin-mediated streptococcal and staphylococcal disease. *J Am Acad Dermatol* 1998;39:383–398.

63. Wermers RA, Fatourechi V, Wynne AG, et al. The glucagonoma syndrome. Clinical and pathologic features in 21 patients. *Medicine (Baltimore)* 1996;75:53–63.

64. Kasper CS. Necrolytic migratory erythema: unresolved problems in diagnosis and pathogenesis. A case report and literature review. *Cutis* 1992;49:120–128.

65. Leichter SB. Clinical and metabolic aspects of glucagonoma. *Medicine (Baltimore)* 1980;59:100–113.

66. Macey WH. A primary care approach to cutaneous T-cell lymphoma. *Nurse Pract.* 2000;25:82, 85–88, 91–94.
67. Basler RS, Lynch PJ. Mycosis fungoides: clinical and therapeutic review. *J Fam Pract* 1979;8:281–286.
68. Basler RS, Lynch PJ. Can you recognize and treat mycosis fungoides? *Geriatrics* 1978;33:55–62.
69. Wong TY, Mihm MC Jr. Images in clinical medicine. Mycosis fungoides. *N Engl J Med* 1993;329:2001.
70. Wolf R, Ruocco V. Triggered psoriasis. *Adv Exp Med Biol* 1999;455:221–225.
71. Abel EA. Diagnosis of drug-induced psoriasis. *Semin Dermatol* 1992;11:269–274.
72. Abel EA, DiCicco LM, Orenberg EK, et al. Drugs in exacerbation of psoriasis. *J Am Acad Dermatol* 1986;15:1007–1022.
73. Pawlotsky JM, Dhumeaux D, Bagot M. Hepatitis C virus in dermatology. A review [see comments]. *Arch Dermatol* 1995; 131:1185–1193.
74. Massi D, Borgognoni L, Franchi A, et al. Thick cutaneous malignant melanoma: a reappraisal of prognostic factors. *Melanoma Res* 2000;10:153–164.
75. Case records of the Massachusetts General Hospital. Weekly clinicopathological exercises. Case 7-1999. A 50-year-old woman with severe diarrhea during radiation treatment for resected metastatic melanoma [clinical conference]. *N Engl J Med* 1999;340:789–796.
76. Lotti T, Ghersetich I, Comacchi C, et al. Cutaneous small-vessel vasculitis. *J Am Acad Dermatol* 1998;39:667–687.
77. Ekenstam E, Callen JP. Cutaneous leukocytoclastic vasculitis. Clinical and laboratory features of 82 patients seen in private practice. *Arch Dermatol* 1984;120:484–489.
78. Gorevic PD, Kassab HJ, Levo Y, et al. Mixed cryoglobulinemia: clinical aspects and long-term follow-up of 40 patients. *Am J Med* 1980;69:287–308.
79. Blanco R, Martinez-Taboada VM, Rodriguez-Valverde V, et al. Cutaneous vasculitis in children and adults. Associated diseases and etiologic factors in 303 patients. *Medicine (Baltimore)* 1998;77:403–418.
80. Farrell AM, Dawber RP. Sign of Leser-Trelat [Letter; comment]. *J Am Acad Dermatol* 1997;37:138–139.
81. Schwartz RA. Sign of Leser-Trelat [see comments]. *J Am Acad Dermatol* 1996;35:88–95.

4

ENDOCRINOLOGY

1. Most **thyroid function test** abnormalities newly diagnosed in the hospital will normalize when retested as an outpatient (1).

2. **Addison disease** (primary adrenal insufficiency) should be suspected with hypotension that is refractory to fluid resuscitation (2,3).

3. Postpartum endocrinopathy, including amenorrhea, lack of lactation, hypothyroidism, and adrenal insufficiency, suggests **Sheehan syndrome** (peripartum pituitary apoplexy) (4).

4. The combination of exophthalmos, thyroid acropachy, and pretibial myxedema are pathognomonic for **Graves disease**. Exophthalmos is proptosis, ophthalmoplegia, and ocular congestion, whereas thyroid acropachy is clubbing of the fingers and toes with painless bony changes. Pretibial myxedema is a peau d'orange on the dorsum of the legs that is classically nonpitting (5,6).

5. Remember the possibility of **myxedema coma** when facing an unresponsive patient who has a healed neck scar (7).

6. Patients with **acromegaly** may present with increased hand, foot, hat size, and prognathism. Other more subtle findings can include tongue enlargement, with tooth marks on the tongue; wide spacing of the teeth; coarse facial features; obstructive sleep apnea; new onset hypertension; carpal tunnel syndrome; arthralgias involving shoulders, back, and knees; hollow-sounding voice from laryngeal and sinus hypertrophy;

congestive heart failure; goiter; increased skin tags; doughy handshake; and oily skin (8,9).

7. **Pheochromocytoma** classically presents with paroxysmal or continuous hypertension, episodic palpitations, headaches, tremor, chest pain, and pallor. Note that flushing is unusual in pheochromocytoma and should suggest an alternative diagnosis (10).

8. **Hyperaldosteronism** should be sought in any patient who presents with hypertension and hypokalemia. These patients are typically not hypernatremic because both sodium and water are reabsorbed from the distal convoluted tubule (11,12).

9. One question to distinguish **osteoporosis** versus **osteomalacia** is the presence of bone pain. In the absence of a bone fracture, osteoporosis is a painless disease. Osteomalacia, on the other hand, is classically associated with dull, aching bone pain. Laboratory abnormalities associated with osteomalacia are hypophosphatemia (renal tubular wasting and vitamin D deficiency), hypocalcemia (vitamin D deficiency), and elevated alkaline phosphatase. Primary osteoporosis is not associated with laboratory abnormalities (13–15).

10. Patients with **primary aldosteronism** usually do not have edema despite having an expanded extracellular fluid volume (12).

11. Hypokalemic alkalosis is a major manifestation of ectopic **production** of corticotropin. Classic features of Cushing syndrome are often absent (16).

12. Hyperpigmentation in a patient with **Cushing syndrome** points to an extraadrenal tumor, either intracranial or ectopic (16–18).

13. Diabetes mellitus (DM) and amyloidosis are two diseases that should come to mind when patients present with signs of **autonomic insufficiency**: delayed gastric emptying, diarrhea, orthostatic hypotension, brady- or tachyarrhythmias, and bladder dysfunction (19–21).

14. Elderly patients who present with depression may have **apathetic hyperthyroidism**. One clue to this disease process is the combination of recently diagnosed depression coincident with new-onset atrial fibrillation (22).

15. The most common causes of thyrotoxicosis with a **low neck radioiodine uptake (RAIU)** are thyroiditis (subacute or postpartum), factitious from exogenous ingestion of thyroid hormones, excessive thyroid replacement, and ectopic thyroid tissue (struma ovarii) (23).

16. The common causes of thyrotoxicosis with a **high neck RAIU** are Graves disease, toxic multinodular goiter, and autonomously functioning thyroid nodule. Less common causes are thyrotropin-secreting pituitary tumor and excessive β-HCG production (tumors, molar pregnancy) (24).

17. A patient undergoing surgical removal of a **pheochromocytoma** should have preoperative administration of both an α-blocker and a β-blocker. The danger of administering only a β-blocker to prevent intraoperative hypertension is the possibility of unopposed alpha stimulation. This can lead to overwhelming vasoconstriction, severe hypertension, cardiac ischemia, and pulmonary edema (25).

18. Calcifications seen on head computed tomography scan in the basal ganglia and cerebellum in a patient with a history of paresthesia, tetany, and seizures suggest the diagnosis of **hypoparathyroidism** (26,27).

19. **Hirsutism** refers specifically to excessive growth of androgen-dependent hair, whereas **virilization** refers to general development of male secondary sex characteristics, including clitoromegaly, hirsutism, male-pattern balding, acne, and deepening of the voice. Excessive androgen production typically arises from the ovary, adrenal gland, or exogenously. One way to distinguish adrenal androgen production from ovarian androgen excess is the serum dehydroepiandrosterone-S (DHEA-S) level, which is often elevated in cases of adrenal androgen excess (28,29).

20. Most **thyroid nodules** are benign. It is important to note that thyroid cancer occurs at a similar frequency whether it arises from a multinodular goiter or an isolated solitary nodule (30).

21. The diagnosis of **Paget disease** should be suggested in patients who have an isolated elevation in their alkaline phosphatase with normal liver function tests and a serum calcium. Most patients with Paget disease are asymptomatic. The most common clinical manifestations are focal bone pain and skeletal deformity. Detecting an elevated alkaline phosphatase and then demonstrating pagetic bone on plain films usually confirms the diagnosis. The most common complication is bone fracture; the feared complication is osteogenic sarcoma (31).

22. Primary hyperparathyroidism is often associated with a hyperchloremic metabolic acidosis, a finding that is not usually associated with hypercalcemia of malignancy. **Serum chloride** level may be a rough way of differentiating between primary hyperparathyroidism and hypercalcemia of malignancy, although not a substitute for serum parathyroid hormone (PTH) and PTHrp (32,33).

23. The possibility of **rhinocerebral mucormycosis** should be entertained in a patient who presents with diabetic ketoacidosis and has persistent mental status change after correction of fluid and electrolyte disturbances. Most patients complain of headache, facial pain, epistaxis, or visual impairment, depending on the location of fungal invasion. Proptosis can be seen on physical examination. Mucormycosis is an angioinvasive fungus that can lead to cerebrovascular accidents (34,35).

24. The most common location for **corticotropin-producing tumors** is the pituitary gland. However, in patients with corticotropin-dependent Cushing's syndrome, it is important to perform a high dose dexamethasone suppression test to prove the pituitary origin of corticotropin. This should be done before imaging for a pituitary adenoma, because non-

functioning but radiographically visible pituitary adenomas are common (36).

25. A patient who presents with mucosal neuromas on the lips and tongue should be genetically screened for **multiple endocrine neoplasia type 2B**, an autosomal-dominant disease characterized by marfanoid body habitus, mucosal neuromas, dysmorphic facies, and, most importantly, pheochromocytoma and medullary thyroid carcinoma (37).

26. A **neuroendocrine tumor VIPoma** (vasoactive intestinal polypeptide) should be considered in a patient who presents with watery diarrhea typically greater than 3 L/day that persists with fasting accompanied by hypokalemia, achlorhydria, and weight loss. This is a rare disorder, therefore, other forms of secretory diarrhea should be considered: infectious enteritis, collagenous colitis, laxative abuse, inflammatory bowel disease, villous adenoma, hyperthyroidism, carcinoid syndrome, and ileal resection (bile malabsorption) (38).

27. Patients who present with **diabetes insipidus (DI)** typically have serum sodium values in the upper range of normal. Patients with uncomplicated DI should have intact thirst centers that alert them to increase fluid intake and lower the serum sodium. A patient with underlying DI found to have sodium levels in the 160s clearly has another underlying pathology (e.g., damage to the thirst center) or has no free access water, leading to severe dehydration and hypernatremia (39).

28. An **adrenal incidentaloma** should be surgically removed if it is a functional tumor or malignant. Many experts agree that an adrenal incidentaloma greater than 6 cm and most between 4 and 6 cm should be removed because of the increased likelihood of malignancy. Any adrenal tumor associated with Cushing syndrome, pheochromocytoma, or hyperaldosteronism necessitates surgical removal (40).

29. **Type I diabetic nephropathy** should be seriously questioned in a diabetic with a normal funduscopic

examination. Diabetic retinopathy should precede the development of type I diabetic nephropathy. Less correlation is found between retinopathy and nephropathy in type II DM. Other causes of proteinuria should be investigated in patients with underlying DM if the proteinuria develops within 5 years of the initial diagnosis of diabetes, or if the urine sediment shows active white blood cells, red blood cell casts, or white blood cell casts. Diabetic nephropathy should be accompanied by a bland sediment (41).

30. **Thyroid storm** should be considered in a patient with exaggerated features of hyperthyroidism. These patients often have a preexisting diagnosis of thyroid disease. Hyperpyrexia with temperatures well above 104°F, significant tachycardia, atrial fibrillation, congestive heart failure, severe diarrhea, delirium, seizures, or jaundice can accompany thyroid storm. It most commonly occurs after surgery or after receiving a substantial iodine load (42).

31. A patient who presents with progressive centripetal obesity (affecting the face, neck, trunk, and abdomen, but sparing extremities) should be worked up for **Cushing syndrome**. Other findings include: easy bruisability, purple striae, worsening hypertension or diabetes, myopathic weakness, and increased susceptibility to infections (18).

32. Hypotension (resting or orthostatic), abdominal pain, anorexia, or vomiting after initiating thyroid hormone replacement, in a patient with preexisting hypothyroidism, suggests **coexistent adrenal insufficiency** (43,44).

33. The concern for patients who present with a **thyroid nodule** is whether it is malignant. Three groups have an increased risk of malignant nodules: adult patients less than 30 and those greater than 60 years of age, children, and patients with a history of head or neck irradiation (45).

34. Preeclampsia in the first trimester of pregnancy should indicate a diagnosis of **gestational trophoblastic disease** (i.e., hydatidiform mole) (46).

35. The differential diagnosis of unintentional **weight loss** with a preserved appetite is short: DM, hyperthyroidism, and malabsorption syndromes. Patients who lose weight secondary to malignancies, inflammatory diseases, infectious diseases, and depression tend to have poor appetites (47,48).

36. **Diabetes insipidus** in a patient with a sellar mass strongly suggests that the patient does not have a pituitary adenoma, because less than 1% of patients with pituitary adenomas have DI. More likely causes include hypothalamic disease (i.e., sarcoidosis, craniopharyngioma, or metastatic breast cancer) (49).

REFERENCES

1. Attia J, Margetts P, Guyatt G. Diagnosis of thyroid disease in hospitalized patients: a systematic review [see comments]. *Arch Intern Med* 1999;159:658–665.
2. Keljo DJ, Squires RH Jr. Clinical problem-solving. Just in time [see comments]. *N Engl J Med* 1996;334:46–48.
3. Chin R. Adrenal crisis. *Crit Care Clin* 1991;7:23–42.
4. Vance ML. Hypopituitarism [published erratum appears in *N Engl J Med* 1994;331(7):487]. *N Engl J Med* 1994;330: 1651–1662.
5. Dabon-Almirante CL, Surks MI. Clinical and laboratory diagnosis of thyrotoxicosis. *Endocrinol Metab Clin North Am* 1998; 27:25–35.
6. Bahn RS, Heufelder AE. Pathogenesis of Graves' ophthalmopathy. *N Engl J Med* 1993;329:1468–1475.
7. Martinez FJ, Lash RW. Endocrinologic and metabolic complications in the intensive care unit. *Clin Chest Med* 1999;20: 401–421, ix.
8. Melmed S. Acromegaly [see comments]. *N Engl J Med* 1990; 322:966–977.
9. Nabarro JD. Acromegaly. *Clin Endocrinol (Oxf)* 1987;26: 481–512.
10. Young WF Jr, Maddox DE. Spells: in search of a cause. *Mayo Clin Proc* 1995;70:757–765.
11. Ganguly A. Primary aldosteronism. *N Engl J Med* 1998;339: 1828–1834.
12. Gregoire JR. Adjustment of the osmostat in primary aldosteronism. *Mayo Clin Proc* 1994;69:1108–1110.
13. Hurley DL, Khosla S. Update on primary osteoporosis. *Mayo Clin Proc* 1997;72:943–949.

14. Reginato AJ, Falasca GF, Pappu R, et al. Musculoskeletal manifestations of osteomalacia: report of 26 cases and literature review. *Semin Arthritis Rheum* 1999;28:287–304.

15. Bingham CT, Fitzpatrick LA. Noninvasive testing in the diagnosis of osteomalacia [see comments]. *Am J Med* 1993;95:519–523.

16. Delisle L, Boyer MJ, Warr D, et al. Ectopic corticotropin syndrome and small-cell carcinoma of the lung. Clinical features, outcome, and complications. *Arch Intern Med* 1993;153:746–752.

17. Agarwala SS. Paraneoplastic syndromes. *Med Clin North Am* 1996;80:173–184.

18. Orth DN. Cushing's syndrome [published erratum appears in N Engl J Med 1995;332(22):1527]. *N Engl J Med* 1995;332:791–803.

19. Watkins PJ. Diabetic autonomic neuropathy [editorial, comment]. *N Engl J Med* 1990;322:1078–1079.

20. DiSalvo TG, King ME, Smith RN. Case records of the Massachusetts General Hospital. Weekly clinicopathological exercises. Case 3-2000. A 66-year-old woman with diabetes, coronary disease, orthostatic hypotension and the nephrotic syndrome [clinical conference]. *N Engl J Med* 2000;342:264–273.

21. Rajkumar SV, Gertz MA, Kyle RA. Prognosis of patients with primary systemic amyloidosis who present with dominant neuropathy. *Am J Med* 1998;104:232–237.

22. Levy EG. Thyroid disease in the elderly. *Med Clin North Am* 1991;75:151–167.

23. Ross DS. Syndromes of thyrotoxicosis with low radioactive iodine uptake. *Endocrinol Metab Clin North Am* 1998;27:169–185.

24. Summaria V, Salvatori M, Rufini V, et al. Diagnostic imaging in thyrotoxicosis. *Rays (Milano)* 1999;24:273–300.

25. Werbel SS, Ober KP. Pheochromocytoma. Update on diagnosis, localization, and management. *Med Clin North Am* 1995;79:131–153.

26. Polverosi R, Zambelli C, Sbeghen R. Calcification of the basal nuclei in hypoparathyroidism. The computed and magnetic resonance tomographic aspects. *Radiol Med (Torino)* 1994;87:12–15.

27. Sanchetee P, Venkataraman S, Mohan C, et al. Basal ganglia calcification. *J Assoc Physicians India* 1999;47:507–509.

28. Case records of the Massachusetts General Hospital. Weekly clinicopathological exercises. Case 24-1993. A

56-year-old woman with virilization. *N Engl J Med* 1993;328: 1770–1776.

29. Ehrmann DA, Rosenfield RL. Hirsutism–beyond the steroidogenic block [editorial]. *N Engl J Med* 1990;323: 909–911.

30. Case records of the Massachusetts General Hospital. Weekly clinicopathological exercises. Case 44-1986. An 80-year-old woman with Paget's disease and severe hypercalcemia after a recent fracture. *N Engl J Med* 1986;315:1209–1219.

31. Delmas PD, Meunier PJ. The management of Paget's disease of bone. *N Engl J Med* 1987;20,336:558–566.

32. Lind L, Ljunghall S. Serum chloride in the differential diagnosis of hypercalcemia. *Exp Clin Endocrinol* 19991;98:179–184.

33. Broulik PD, Pacovsky V. The chloride phosphate ratio as the screening test for primary hyperparathyroidism. *Horm Metab Res* 1979;11:577–579.

34. Rupp ME. Images in clinical medicine. Rhinocerebral mucormycosis. *N Engl J Med* 1995;333:564.

35. Butugan O, Sanchez TG, Goncalez F, et al. Rhinocerebral mucormycosis: predisposing factors, diagnosis, therapy, complications and survival. *Rev Laryngol Otol Rhinol (Bord)* 1996; 117:53–55.

36. Grua JR, Nelson DH. ACTH-producing pituitary tumors. *Endocrinol Metab Clin North Am* 1991;20:319–362.

37. Raue F, Zink A. Clinical features of multiple endocrine neoplasia type 1 and type 2. *Horm Res* 1992;38 [Suppl 2]:31–35.

38. Krejs GJ. VIPoma syndrome. *Am J Med* 1987;82:37–48.

39. Adam P. Evaluation and management of diabetes insipidus. *Am Fam Physician* 1997;55:2146–2153.

40. Kievit J, Haak HR. Diagnosis and treatment of adrenal incidentaloma. A cost-effectiveness analysis. *Endocrinol Metab Clin North Am* 2000;29:69–ix.

41. Parving HH, Hommel E, Mathiesen E, et al. Prevalence of microalbuminuria, arterial hypertension, retinopathy and neuropathy in patients with insulin dependent diabetes. *BMJ (Clinical Research Ed)* 1988;296:156–160.

42. Mackin JF, Canary JJ, Pittman CS. Thyroid storm and its management. *N Engl J Med* 1974;291:1396–1398.

43. Banitt PF, Munson AK. Addisonian crisis after thyroid replacement. *Hosp Pract (Off Ed)* 1986;21:132, 134.

44. Oelkers W. Adrenal insufficiency [see comments]. *N Engl J Med* 1996;335:1206–1212.

45. Burch HB. Evaluation and management of the solid thyroid nodule. *Endocrinol Metab Clin North Am* 1995;24:663–710.

46. Ramsey PS, Van Winter JT, Gaffey A, et al. Eclampsia complicating hydatidiform molar pregnancy with a coexisting, viable fetus. A case report. *J Reprod Med* 1998;43:456–458.
47. Wise GR, Craig D. Evaluation of involuntary weight loss. Where do you start? *Postgrad Med* 1994;95:143–150.
48. Reife CM. Involuntary weight loss. *Med Clin North Am* 1995; 79:299–313.
49. Freda PU, Post KD. Differential diagnosis of sellar masses. *Endocrinol Metab Clin North Am* 1999;28:81–117, vi.

5

GASTROENTEROLOGY

1. **Mesenteric ischemia** should be considered on the differential diagnosis when abdominal pain is severe and out of proportion to findings on the abdominal examination. The abdominal pain is typically located periumbilically. A mesenteric angiogram should be pursued early if the patient is stable. Endoscopy is of limited value. The most common intestinal sites to be affected by ischemic colitis are the watershed territories (areas that lie between major blood vessels) of the splenic flexure and the sigmoid colon. The rectum is usually spared because of its dual blood supply (1,2).

2. Multiple, recurrent gastrointestinal (GI) ulcers, especially when located beyond the duodenum, (i.e., jejunal ulcers) associated with diarrhea suggest **Zollinger-Ellison syndrome** (3).

3. **Aminotransferases greater than 1,000** U/L are associated with viral hepatitis, toxin, drug, or ischemic injury. Drug-induced fulminant liver failure carries a poor prognosis, with the exception of acetaminophen-induced hepatic injury wherein most patients recover (4).

4. Alcohol rarely causes aminotransferase elevation greater than 500 U/L. The **aspartate aminotransferase-to-alanine aminotransferase (ASP:ALT) ratio** is usually greater than **2:1** (5).

5. Patients with repeated bouts of what appears clinically to be an **acute abdomen** may have abdominal pain of metabolic origin. Oftentimes, these patients will have preexisting RLQ surgical scars from negative laparoscopic workup. The differential diagnosis

should include acute intermittent porphyria, familial Mediterranean fever, C1 esterase deficiency associated with hereditary angioneurotic edema, lead poisoning, diabetic ketoacidosis, black widow spider bite, and vasculitides (e.g., polyarteritis nodosa) (6–9).

6. **Celiac sprue** should be considered high on the differential diagnosis of malabsorptive diarrhea, especially when associated with iron deficiency anemia refractory to iron supplementation, or hypocalcemia, which can lead to osteomalacia (10,11).

7. The triad of alopecia, desquamating skin lesions of the perioral or perianal areas, and diarrhea should raise concern for **acrodermatitis enteropathica**, a disease of zinc malabsorption. Impaired dark adaptation because of decreased vitamin A conversion can occur. Treatment with zinc sulfate orally may produce a dramatic recovery (12).

8. The greater the lipase-to-amylase ratio (**Tenner-Steinberg**) in acute pancreatitis (greater than 2:1), the more likely it is caused by alcohol abuse as opposed to gallstones (13).

9. Hemolysis complicating otherwise unexplained liver disease in a young adult suggests **Wilson disease**. High red blood cell copper released from the liver causes hemolysis. The alkaline phosphatase is disproportionately lower than the other aminotransferases. Another clue may be low serum uric acid levels (14,15).

10. Once it has been confirmed that a patient is having **diarrhea** (greater than 200 g/day), the next question is whether the diarrhea lessens with fasting. Diarrhea that decreases with fasting is osmotically mediated. Diarrhea persisting on fasting is either secretory or inflammatory. Many patients with chronic diarrhea have irritable bowel syndrome, a form of GI dysmotility. These patients sleep through the night without diarrhea (16).

11. **Whipple disease** is a rare cause of chronic abdominal pain, diarrhea, weight loss, and arthralgias. The

most common host is a middle-aged man of European descent. Other less common features are polyarthritis, hyperpigmentation, fevers, lymphadenopathy, and central nervous system (CNS) abnormalities. It should be considered in the differential of fever of unknown origin (FUO), polyserositis, generalized adenopathy, polyarthritis, and encephalopathy (17,18).

12. **Primary sclerosing cholangitis (PSC)** is a chronic autoimmune liver disease that leads to strictures of intra- and extrahepatic bile ducts. It typically affects men with liver function test results that show a disproportionate elevation in alkaline phosphatase and bilirubin as compared with aminotransferases. A close association is found between PSC and inflammatory bowel disease. Of patients with primary sclerosing cholangitis, 70% have underlying ulcerative colitis. However, patients with ulcerative colitis only have a 5% chance of acquiring PSC (19).

13. Fever in a cirrhotic patient with ascites is **spontaneous bacterial peritonitis** until proved otherwise. A diagnostic paracentesis demonstrating greater than 250 polymorphonuclear cells/mm^3 requires the patient have antibiotic coverage until culture results are available (20).

14. The triad of recurrent epistaxis or GI bleeding, multiple telangiectasias, and family history is diagnostic of hereditary hemorrhagic telangiectasias (HHT), otherwise known as **Osler-Weber-Rendu disease**. The complications of this disease include life-threatening GI bleeding, massive pulmonary hemorrhage, and paradoxical emboli from pulmonary atriovenous malformations, leading to cerebrovascular accidents. Patients with HHT are also at higher risk of septic emboli leading to brain abscesses. Recurrent epistaxis and telangiectasias of the tongue are often the first manifestation of the disease, occurring in the first decade of life, whereas the cutaneous telangiectasias do not classically present until the second or third decade (21–23).

15. The diagnosis of **tropical sprue** should be entertained in a patient who has chronic diarrhea, weight loss, megaloblastic anemia, and other stigmata of malabsorption (cheilitis, vitamin D deficiency, or hypocalcemia), and has spent greater than 2 weeks in a country endemic with tropical sprue. Folate replacement can improve symptoms dramatically to the point where clinical response to folate can be used as a diagnostic aid (24).

16. Dysphagia to both solids and liquids early in the course of the disease should raise suspicion for **achalasia**. This is in contrast to esophageal cancer in which difficulty swallowing solids classically precedes dysphagia to liquids. Achalasia may be primary (most common in the United States) or secondary to gastric cancer invading the esophagus, lymphoma, or Chagas disease. Gastroesophageal reflux disease argues against achalasia. Diagnosis is usually made with a barium swallow, which shows a beaklike narrowing of the terminal esophagus representing the nonrelaxing lower esophageal sphincter. Manometry may demonstrate failure of the lower esophageal sphincter to relax in response to swallowing (25).

17. Clues to the presence of the autosomal recessive disease **abetalipoproteinemia** include total cholesterol greater than 50 mg/dl and neurologic stigmata of vitamin E deficiency (e.g., ataxia). Chylomicrons, which are absent in this disease, are required to transport vitamins such as A and E. This disease, more common in children than adults, should be suspected when the patient presents with the triad of chronic diarrhea, ataxia, and hypocholesterolemia (26,27).

18. The combination of chronic abdominal pain and peripheral motor neuropathy in an adult suggests **lead poisoning**. These patients may also have short-term memory loss and difficulty concentrating. One clue on physical examination may be a "lead line" at the tooth-gingiva border. Peripheral blood smear demonstrates red blood cell basophilic stippling.

Lead poisoning in children more commonly presents with peripheral neuropathy, whereas adults have more CNS disease (28).

19. Fatty replacement of the pancreas in a young adult, especially in one who is not obese, should raise suspicion for **cystic fibrosis (CF)**. Obesity can also lead to fatty replacement of the pancreas. It is important to remember that some of these patients with CF may not have a classic history of recurrent sinopulmonary infections, clubbing on physical examination, or bronchiectasis on chest CT (29).

20. **Eosinophilic gastroenteritis** should be considered in any patient who presents with chronic abdominal symptoms and peripheral eosinophilia. It should be noted that peripheral eosinophilia may be absent in the minority of cases. The diagnosis is made by GI tissue biopsy demonstrating increased eosinophils, in the absence of parasitic disease. Symptoms depend on the location of eosinophilic involvement. When disease is limited to the mucosa of the stomach, symptoms such as nausea, vomiting, and abdominal pain may predominate. If the mucosa of the small bowel is affected, a malabsorption syndrome may ensue with iron deficiency anemia and protein-losing enteropathy. Disease that primarily affects the muscularis layer can cause obstructive type symptoms and delayed GI transit. The subserosal layer may be infiltrated with eosinophils and lead to eosinophilic ascites. This is a challenging diagnosis to make in the absence of peripheral eosinophilia (30).

21. **Gilbert syndrome**, a disorder characterized by impaired hepatic uptake of bilirubin, is often first suspected with the discovery of an elevated indirect serum bilirubin in an otherwise healthy patient. These patients should have no other LFT abnormalities and no hemolysis. One clue to this diagnosis is that the indirect hyperbilirubinemia is often more elevated after periods of fasting. Jaundiced skin may result, causing patients to seek medical attention (31).

22. **Oculomasticatory myorhythmia**, continuous rhythmic movement of the eyes along with muscles of mastication, is an uncommon but a pathognomonic finding in Whipple disease (32).

23. In a patient with ascites of unknown cause, a **serum—ascites albumin gradient** greater than 1.1 in ascitic fluid implies portal hypertension with 95% probability (33).

24. Consider the diagnosis of **distal ileal obstructive syndrome** (formerly referred to as "meconium ileus") in otherwise healthy young adults who present with recurrent episodes of small bowel obstruction. This syndrome is caused by CF. Other more common causes of small bowel obstruction [e.g., adhesions, inflammatory bowel disease, malignancies (lymphoma and carcinoid tumor), and hernias] should be ruled out first (34,35).

25. A patient with biopsy-proven celiac sprue positive serology (e.g., antigliadin antibody) who continues to have weight loss and diarrhea despite successful gluten restriction, should be investigated for the possibility of **small bowel T-cell lymphoma**, one of the feared complications of celiac disease (36–38).

26. **Toxic megacolon** should be considered in any patient with underlying inflammatory bowel disease or infectious colitis who presents with high fevers, abdominal pain, rebound tenderness, diarrhea, tachycardia, leukocytosis, altered sensorium, and dilated colon on abdominal plain films (39,40).

27. Four clinical clues of **cirrhosis** distal to the wrist are clubbing, Dupuytren contracture, palmar erythema, and Terry nails. Other features include gynecomastia, testicular atrophy, ascites, caput medusae, and spider angioma (41).

28. It is clear that longstanding inflammatory bowel disease predisposes patients to **colorectal cancer**. The more extensive the degree of colitis, the greater the risk of colorectal cancer. Patients with isolated ulcerative proctitis are at less risk for colorectal cancer than patients with pancolitis (42,43).

29. Consider **infliximab** (anti–TNF-α therapy) for patients with Crohn disease and fistulas (44).

30. The microbiology differs between **spontaneous bacterial peritonitis (SBP)** and **secondary bacterial peritonitis**. The presence of a single aerobic organism suggests SBP, whereas mixed flora (gram-negative rods and anaerobic organisms) are typically seen in secondary bacterial peritonitis (45,46).

31. Patients with moderate to severe Crohn disease undergoing treatment with the immunosuppressive agent **6-mercaptopurine (6-MP)** who present with a Crohn flare should have an erythrocyte 6-MP serum level drawn to ensure a therapeutic level. If the level is low, the dosage may need to be increased (47).

32. **Collagenous colitis** should be suspected in older women who present with features of secretory diarrhea (diarrhea that persists with fasting), features of irritable bowel syndrome (chronic abdominal pain), and features of inflammatory bowel disease (weight loss and presence of fecal leukocytes). Colonoscopy demonstrates normal colonic mucosa but biopsies show a layer of increased subepithelial collagen, and increased lymphocytes in the lamina propria. Right-sided colon biopsies have greater yield than left-sided biopsies; however, left-sided biopsies prove the diagnosis in most patients. "Heme" positive stools make collagenous colitis less likely (48).

33. **Budd-Chiari syndrome** can present acutely, subacutely, or chronically. The acute form should be considered in patients who present with right upper quadrant abdominal pain, hepatomegaly, rapid onset ascites, and jaundice. The subacute or chronic form should be considered in patients who present with unexplained ascites and unexplained hepatomegaly. Females are more likely to develop the acute form of Budd-Chiari, oftentimes with an underlying hypercoagulable state (oral contraception, polycythemia and factor V Leiden mutation) (49).

34. Clues that suggest **alcoholic hepatitis** are a recent history of binge drinking, low grade fever, leukocyto-

sis, transaminitis with an AST-to-ALT ratio greater than 2, jaundice, and tender hepatomegaly. Once other causes for leukocytosis have been ruled out, the greater the elevation of white blood cell count, the greater the amount of hepatocyte injury. AST and ALT elevations greater than 500 U/L should suggest an alternative diagnosis. Rarely, two simultaneous processes could be occurring (e.g., alcoholic hepatitis and acetaminophen toxicity) (50,51).

35. The combination of pruritus, hepatomegaly, hyperpigmentation, and a disproportionately elevated alkaline phosphatase level in a woman above 30 years of age suggests **primary biliary cirrhosis (PBC)** and is uncommon for other liver diseases. Hypercholesterolemia and sicca-type symptoms (dry eyes /dry skin) strengthen the diagnosis. The triad of an elevated alkaline phosphatase, increased total IgM fraction, and positive antimitochondrial antibodies essentially confirms the diagnosis of PBC. Liver biopsy remains the gold standard for the diagnosis of PBC (52).

36. The presence of **Streptococcal bovis endocarditis** or *Clostridium septicum* **bacteremia** suggests GI malignancy and mandates a colonoscopy and endoscopic gastroduodenoscopy (EGD) (53,54).

37. When taken orally, certain pills can lead directly to esophagitis, a condition termed **pill esophagitis**: iron, tetracycline, nonsteroidal antiinflammatory drugs (NSAIDS), bisphosphonates (alendronate), quinidine, and potassium. The clinical presentation often consists of the acute onset of retrosternal chest pain with associated odynophagia. This is particularly true in older patients with esophageal dysmotility (55).

38. A patient who presents with acute pancreatitis and the sudden onset of blindness likely has **Purtscher retinopathy** (56).

39. Normal aminotransferases do **not** rule out **hepatitis C virus (HCV)** in a patient with underlying risk factors for the disease. HCV can occur with normal aminotransferases. Aminotransferases tend to fluctuate

throughout the course of the disease and can be low, normal, or high at any given time (57).

40. **Hyperemesis gravidarum (HG)**, which is seen in the first trimester of pregnancy, is characterized by intractable nausea and vomiting, abnormal liver function tests, and weight loss. Abdominal pain is mild or absent. Hyperthyroidism, a relatively uncommon condition during pregnancy, can mimic HG (58).

41. A number of patients with underlying HCV liver disease have developed fulminant liver failure with subsequent **hepatitis A virus superinfection**. It is important to vaccinate patients against hepatitis A virus if they are infected with HCV (59).

42. In a patient with suspected liver disease, an antinuclear antibody (ANA) of greater than or equal to 1:40 in the absence of viral hepatitis warrants an evaluation for **autoimmune hepatitis** demonstrated by the presence of plasma cell infiltration on liver biopsy. This is an important diagnosis to entertain because treatment with immunosuppressives may reverse the hepatic pathology (60).

43. **Suppurative pylephlebitis** or inflammation of the portal vein secondary to infectious causes should be considered in the differential diagnosis of multiple liver microabscesses. It can arise from ruptured appendicitis, diverticulitis, or, in females, infection of the pelvis. It is most commonly associated with biliary tract disease. Fever is invariable and other symptoms are similar to those seen in liver abscesses. Abdominal computed tomography scan with contrast can show a density in the portal vein that may represent pus or clot in the case of pylethrombophlebitis (61,62).

REFERENCES

1. Bharucha AE, Tremaine WJ, Johnson CD, et al. Ischemic proctosigmoiditis. *Am J Gastroenterol* 1996;91:2305–2309.
2. McKinsey JF, Gewertz BL. Acute mesenteric ischemia. *Surg Clin North Am* 1997;77:307–318.
3. Hirschowitz BI. Zollinger-Ellison syndrome: pathogenesis, diagnosis, and management. *Am J Gastroenterol* 1997;92:44S–48S.

4. Moseley RH. Evaluation of abnormal liver function tests. *Med Clin North Am* 1996;80:887–906.

5. Sherlock S. Alcoholic liver disease [see comments]. *Lancet* 1995;345:227–229.

6. Chen CC, Thajeb P, Lie SK. Acute intermittent porphyria: clinical analysis of nine cases. *Chung Hua I Hsueh Tsa Chih (Taipei)* 1994;54:395–399.

7. Samuels J, Aksentijevich I, Torosyan Y, et al. Familial Mediterranean fever at the millennium. Clinical spectrum, ancient mutations, and a survey of 100 American referrals to the National Institutes of Health. *Medicine (Baltimore)* 1998;77:268–297.

8. Case records of the Massachusetts General Hospital. Weekly clinicopathological exercises. Case 25-1999. A 16-year-old boy with recurrent abdominal pain [clinical conference] [see comments]. *N Engl J Med* 1999;341:593–599.

9. Roy S, Weimersheimer P. Nonoperative causes of abdominal pain. *Surg Clin North Am* 1997;77:1433–1454.

10. Nehra V. New clinical issues in celiac disease. *Gastroenterol Clin North Am* 1998;27:453–465.

11. Branski D, Lerner A, Lebenthal E. Chronic diarrhea and malabsorption. *Pediatr Clin North Am* 1996;43:307–331.

12. Ozturkcan S, Icagasioglu D, Akyol M, et al. A case of acrodermatitis enteropathica. *J Dermatol* 2000;27:475–477.

13. Tenner SM, Steinberg W. The admission serum lipase:amylase ratio differentiates alcoholic from nonalcoholic acute pancreatitis. *Am J Gastroenterol* 1992;87:1755–1758.

14. Kiss JE, Berman D, Van Thiel D. Effective removal of copper by plasma exchange in fulminant Wilson's disease. *Transfusion* 1998;38:327–331.

15. Case records of the Massachusetts General Hospital. Weekly clinicopathological exercises. Case 1-1997. A 23-year-old man with fulminant hepatorenal failure of uncertain cause [clinical conference] [published erratum appears in *N Engl J Med* 1997; 13;336(7):523]. *N Engl J Med* 1997;336:118–125.

16. Donowitz M, Kokke FT, Saidi R. Evaluation of patients with chronic diarrhea [see comments]. *N Engl J Med* 1995;332: 725–729.

17. Fricker EJ, McDonald TJ, Jr. Images in clinical medicine. Tropheryma whippelii. *N Engl J Med* 1996;335:26.

18. Dobbins WO, III. The diagnosis of Whipple's disease [Editorial; comment]. *N Engl J Med* 1995;332:390–392.

19. Lee YM, Kaplan MM. Primary sclerosing cholangitis. *N Engl J Med* 1995;332:924–933.

20. Boixeda D, De Luis DA, Aller R, et al. Spontaneous bacterial peritonitis. Clinical and microbiological study of 233 episodes. *J Clin Gastroenterol* 1996;23:275–279.

21. Case records of the Massachusetts General Hospital. Weekly clinicopathological exercises. Case 7-1997. A 14-year-old girl with recurrent painless rectal bleeding [clinical conference]. *N Engl J Med* 1997;336:641–648.

22. Nicoleau A, Nicoleau CA. Images in clinical medicine. Hereditary hemorrhagic telangiectasia (Osler-Weber-Rendu disease). *N Engl J Med* 1999;340:1800.

23. Guttmacher AE, Marchuk DA, White RI, Jr. Hereditary hemorrhagic telangiectasia [see comments]. *N Engl J Med* 1995; 333:918–924.

24. Case records of the Massachusetts General Hospital. Weekly clinicopathological exercises. Case 15-1990. A 78-year-old woman from the Dominican Republic with chronic diarrhea. *N Engl J Med* 1990;322:1067–1075.

25. Trate DM, Parkman HP, Fisher RS. Dysphagia. Evaluation, diagnosis, and treatment. *Prim Care* 1996;23:417–432.

26. Tanyel MC, Mancano LD. Neurologic findings in vitamin E deficiency. *Am Fam Physician* 1997;55:197–201.

27. Newman RP, Schaefer EJ, Thomas CB, et al. Abetalipoproteinemia and metastatic spinal cord glioblastoma. *Arch Neurol* 1984;41:554–556.

28. Beigel Y, Ostfeld I, Schoenfeld N. Clinical problem-solving. A leading question [see comments]. *N Engl J Med* 1998;339: 827–830.

29. Soyer P, Spelle L, Pelage JP, et al. Cystic fibrosis in adolescents and adults: fatty replacement of the pancreas—CT evaluation and functional correlation. *Radiology* 1999;210: 611–615.

30. Van Dellen RG, Lewis JC. Oral administration of cromolyn in a patient with protein-losing enteropathy, food allergy, and eosinophilic gastroenteritis. *Mayo Clin Proc* 1994;69:441–444.

31. Wright HR, Gear AJ, Morgan RF, et al. Asymptomatic jaundice after fasting: a diagnostic dilemma. *J Emerg Med* 1997;15: 781–784.

32. Louis ED, Lynch T, Kaufmann P, et al. Diagnostic guidelines in central nervous system Whipple's disease [see comments]. *Ann Neurol* 1996;40:561–568.

33. Runyon BA, Montano AA, Akriviadis EA, et al. The serum-ascites albumin gradient is superior to the exudate-transudate concept in the differential diagnosis of ascites. *Ann Intern Med* 1992;117:215–220.

34. Littlewood JM. Cystic fibrosis: gastrointestinal complications. *Br Med Bull* 1992;48:847–859.

35. Westwood AT, Ireland JD, Bowie MD. Surgery in cystic fibrosis—a 20-year review. *S Afr J Surg* 1997;35:181–184.

36. Egan LJ, Stevens FM, McCarthy CF. Celiac disease and T-cell lymphoma [Letter; comment]. *N Engl J Med* 1996;335: 1611–1612.

37. Case records of the Massachusetts General Hospital. Weekly clinicopathological exercises. Case 15-1996. A 79-year-old woman with anorexia, weight loss, and diarrhea after treatment for celiac disease [clinical conference] [see comments]. *N Engl J Med* 1996;334:1316–1322.

38. Egan LJ, Walsh SV, Stevens FM, et al. Celiac-associated lymphoma. A single institution experience of 30 cases in the combination chemotherapy era. *J Clin Gastroenterol* 1995; 21:123–129.

39. Case records of the Massachusetts General Hospital. Weekly clinicopathological exercises. Case 36-1997. A 58-year-old man with recurrent ulcerative colitis, bloody diarrhea, and abdominal distention [clinical conference]. *N Engl J Med* 1997;337:1532–1540.

40. Heppell J, Farkouh E, Dube S, et al. Toxic megacolon. An analysis of 70 cases. *Dis Colon Rectum* 1986;29:789–792.

41. Hamberg KJ, Carstensen B, Sorensen TI, et al. Accuracy of clinical diagnosis of cirrhosis among alcohol-abusing men. *J Clin Epidemiol* 1996;49:1295–1301.

42. Greenstein AJ. Cancer in inflammatory bowel disease. *Mt Sinai J Med* 2000;67:227–240.

43. Lewis JD, Deren JJ, Lichtenstein GR. Cancer risk in patients with inflammatory bowel disease. *Gastroenterol Clin North Am* 1999;28:459–77, x.

44. Present DH, Rutgeerts P, Targan S, et al. Infliximab for the treatment of fistulas in patients with Crohn's disease. *N Engl J Med* 1999;340:1398–1405.

45. Akriviadis EA, Runyon BA. Utility of an algorithm in differentiating spontaneous from secondary bacterial peritonitis [see comments]. *Gastroenterology* 1990;98:127–133.

46. Guarner C, Soriano G. Spontaneous bacterial peritonitis. *Semin Liver Dis* 1997;17:203–217.

47. Cuffari C, Theoret Y, Latour S, et al. 6-Mercaptopurine metabolism in Crohn's disease: correlation with efficacy and toxicity. *Gut* 1996;39:401–406.

48. Tremaine WJ. Collagenous colitis and lymphocytic colitis. *J Clin Gastroenterol* 2000;30:245–249.

49. Singh V, Sinha SK, Nain CK, et al. Budd-Chiari syndrome: our experience of 71 patients. *J Gastroenterol Hepatol* 2000; 15:550–554.

50. Pratt DS, Kaplan MM. Evaluation of abnormal liver-enzyme results in asymptomatic patients. *N Engl J Med* 2000;342: 1266–1271.

51. Walsh K, Alexander G. Alcoholic liver disease. *Postgrad Med J* 2000;76, 280–286.
52. Kaplan MM. Primary biliary cirrhosis [see comments]. *N Engl J Med* 1996;335:1570–1580.
53. Murray HW, Roberts RB. Streptococcus bovis bacteremia and underlying gastrointestinal disease. *Arch Intern Med* 1978;138:1097–1099.
54. Lorimer JW, Eidus LB. Invasive *Clostridium septicum* infection in association with colorectal carcinoma. *Can J Surg* 1994;37:245–249.
55. Jaspersen D. Drug-induced oesophageal disorders: pathogenesis, incidence, prevention and management. *Drug Saf* 2000;22:237–249.
56. Toshniwal PK, Berman AA, Axelrod AJ. Purtscher's retinopathy secondary to pancreatitis. Aspects of the topography of retinal abnormalities. *J Clin Neuroophthalmol* 1986;6:160–165.
57. Dienstag JL. Management of chronic hepatitis C: a consensus. *Gastroenterology* 1997;113:375.
58. Hod M, Orvieto R, Kaplan B, et al. Hyperemesis gravidarum. A review. *J Reprod Med* 1994;39:605–612.
59. Vento S, Garofano T, Renzini C, et al. Fulminant hepatitis associated with hepatitis A virus superinfection in patients with chronic hepatitis C [see comments]. *N Engl J Med* 1998;338: 286–290.
60. Krawitt EL. Autoimmune hepatitis [see comments]. *N Engl J Med* 1996;334:897–903.
61. Drabick JJ, Landry FJ. Suppurative pylephlebitis. *South Med J* 1991;84:1396–1398.
62. Waxman BP, Cavanagh LL, Nayman J. Suppurative pyephlebitis and multiple hepatic abscesses with silent colonic diverticulitis. *Med J Aust* 1979;2:376–378.

6

HEMATOLOGY

1. An isolated erythrocytosis and palpable spleen represent **polycythemia vera** until proved otherwise (1).

2. Clinically, **massive splenomegaly** is defined as a spleen that extends greater than 8 cm below the left costal margin or one that weighs greater than 1,000 g. Massive splenomegaly is an important finding because it limits the differential diagnosis to the myeloproliferative disorders (MPD) [chronic myelogenous leukemia (CML), polycythemia vera, myelofibrosis with myeloid metaplasia], lymphomas, hairy cell leukemia, Gaucher disease, chronic lymphocytic leukemia (CLL), sarcoidosis, thalassemias, schistosomiasis, or autoimmune hemolytic anemia. It should be noted that portal hypertension from cirrhosis does not lead to massive splenomegaly (2–8).

3. Consider the diagnosis of **systemic mastocytosis** in any patient with an underlying chronic pruritic, urticarial rash associated with flushing, diarrhea, peptic ulcer disease, osteoporosis, organomegaly, or hypotension precipitated by intraoperative anesthesia, nonsteroidal antiinflammatory drugs, or opiates. The skin of patients with systemic mastocytosis may elicit a wheal when rubbed termed "Darier sign" (9).

4. **Microangiopathic hemolytic anemia (MAHA)** on peripheral blood smear is helpful because it narrows the differential diagnosis of anemia. Culprits include disseminated intravascular coagulopathy; hemolytic-uremic syndrome; thrombotic thrombocytopenic purpura (TTP); scleroderma renal crisis; preeclampsia-associated hemolysis, elevated liver

enzymes, low platelets (HELLP syndrome); malignant hypertension; giant cavernous hemangioma (Kasabach-Merritt); and prosthetic valve-associated MAHA (10,11).

5. A middle-aged patient with underlying **hemochromatosis** who is treated with regular phlebotomies to reduce the iron overload, who begins to require fewer phlebotomies should be screened for gastrointestinal (GI) bleeding, in particular a GI malignancy (12).

6. A factor V level may be helpful in a patient who presents with abnormal **bleeding of unknown etiology** because it is the only clotting factor that is produced by the liver that is not vitamin K-dependent and, therefore, if low is an excellent marker for liver disease (13).

7. The diagnosis of **myelofibrosis with myeloid metaplasia**, an MPD, can only be made in the presence of documented bone marrow fibrosis, a leukoerythroblastic peripheral blood smear characterized by nucleated red blood cells, early white blood cell forms, and teardrop red blood cells. Massive splenomegaly is the rule and other MPD should be excluded including CML, polycythemia vera, and essential thrombocythemia. The bone marrow biopsy is essential not only to demonstrate fibrosis, but also to prove the absence of metastatic tumor, infection, connective tissue disease, and myelodysplastic syndrome (normal cytogenetics) (14).

8. The diagnosis of **mixed essential cryoglobulinemia** is made by clinical history (constitutional symptoms, arthralgias, lower extremity palpable purpura, Raynaud phenomenon, and hematuria with renal insufficiency), laboratory abnormalities (hypocomplementemia often with C4 disproportionately diminished), and circulating cryoglobulins. A strong association is seen with hepatitis C virus (HCV) and mixed essential cryoglobulinemia, and the presence of HCV should always be investigated because treatment can be targeted against HCV with antivirals (15).

9. The pentad of tender hepatomegaly, jaundice, ascites, hyperbilirubinemia, and weight gain within

21 days of bone marrow transplantation should suggest the diagnosis of **veno-occlusive disease (VOD)**, a clinical presentation not dissimilar to Budd-Chiari syndrome. The differential diagnosis includes graft-versus-host disease, cholestasis of sepsis, and recurrent malignancy. VOD is often a clinical diagnosis, although transjugular liver biopsy can assist in the diagnosis demonstrating hepatic venular occlusion and centrilobular hemorrhagic necrosis (16).

10. A neutropenic patient that presents with right lower quadrant abdominal pain, fever, and bloody diarrhea should raise suspicion for **typhlitis** (necrotizing colitis, cecal inflammation). Typhlitis most commonly arises in neutropenic patients who have been treated for hematologic malignancies with cytotoxic agents. Rebound tenderness may be present on physical examination and computed tomography (CT) scan is a sensitive means of demonstrating thickening of the cecum. Treatment should begin with antibiotics targeted against gram-negative rods and anaerobes (typical mixed bowel flora). Surgery is occasionally necessary in severe cases (17).

11. **POEMS syndrome** is an acronym for a disease in which the predominant findings are polyneuropathy (sensorimotor), organomegaly (hepatosplenomegaly and lymphadenopathy), endocrinopathy (amenorrhea, decreased libido, diabetes mellitus, hypothyroidism, or hypoadrenalism), M-spike, and skin changes (hyperpigmentation, hypertrichosis, and clubbing). This syndrome has features of both multiple myeloma (M-spike and sclerotic bone lesions) and Waldenstrom macroglobulinemia (organomegaly and a demyelinating polyneuropathy) in addition to the dermatologic and endocrinologic manifestations (18).

12. In a patient with **angioedema**, the presence of a normal C4 level rules out the possibility of hereditary angioneurotic edema (HANE) because the defect is in C1 esterase inhibitor (low levels or dysfunctional) leading to C4 degradation. If the C4 level is low, then C1 esterase inhibitor levels and functional activity

should be assessed in addition to C1q levels. C1q levels are normal in HANE but decreased in acquired C1 esterase inhibitor deficiency. Acquired C1 esterase inhibitor deficiency has been associated with malignancy, in particular B-cell lymphoma (19).

13. A hypogammaglobulinemic patient who develops anaphylaxis after receiving intravenous immunoglobulin (IVIG) should be investigated for **immunoglobulin A (IgA) deficiency**. These patients have anti-IgA antibodies that react with IgA in the IVIG preparation. To combat this life-threatening reaction, IVIG preparations should be used with the lowest possible IgA content (20).

14. Multiple myeloma is one of the causes of a **low** or negative **anion gap** because the monoclonal proteins are cationic (21).

15. A patient who is treated for idiopathic thrombocytopenic purpura (ITP) with IVIG and subsequently develops renal failure may have **IVIG-associated nephrotoxicity** (22).

16. The triad of hemolytic anemia, aplastic anemia, and venous thrombosis (particularly the intraabdominal veins) suggests **paroxysmal nocturnal hemoglobinuria**. Hemoglobinuria reflects the intravascular hemolysis. The unusual combination of bone marrow aplasia and hemolysis is a clue to this rare diagnosis (23).

17. **Thromboangiitis obliterans** (Buerger disease) should be suspected in patients less than 45 years of age who present with forearm, calf, or foot claudication. Men are affected more frequently than women and, although the cause is unknown, smoking appears to be the most important risk factor. Tobacco cessation is the most important treatment modality. Physical examination usually reveals reduced or absent pulses as opposed to antiphospholipid antibody syndrome or cholesterol emboli syndrome where pulses are typically present (24,25).

18. Patients with **Trousseau syndrome**, a superficial migratory thrombophlebitis associated with malig-

nancy, are often resistant to anticoagulation with coumadin and require heparinization to prevent further thromboses (26–28).

19. **Disseminated intravascular coagulation** is one of the serious consequences of acute promyelocytic leukemia (M3 type of acute myelogenous leukemia), whereas **meningeal infiltration** is more common with acute monocytic or myelomonocytic leukemia (M4 and M5) (29,30).

20. The diagnosis of **antiphospholipid antibody syndrome** should be made in patients who present with recurrent venous or arterial thromboses, thrombocytopenia, recurrent fetal loss (classically second trimester), or livedo reticularis. Laboratory findings critical to the diagnosis should be confirmed on two occasions at least 3 months apart: IgM or IgG anticardiolipin antibody, lupus anticoagulant, or anti-B2-glycoprotein I (31).

21. **Hypertrophy** of the **gums** may be secondary to chronic phenytoin, cyclosporin, or nifedipine use as well as from leukemic infiltration in acute myelomonocytic leukemia (32,33).

22. **Microangiopathic hemolytic anemia** should be suspected in a patient who presents with a nonimmune hemolysis (negative Coombs test) combined with a peripheral blood smear that demonstrates schistocytes and helmet cells. The red blood cells are fragmented to such a degree that the mean corpuscular volume may be reduced. In a nonpregnant patient, MAHA and thrombocytopenia should raise suspicion for TTP or hemolytic uremic syndrome. An elevated lactate dehydrogenase level is typically present with MAHA and can be used, in addition to serial hematocrits, to judge the severity of the anemia (10,11).

23. **Catastrophic antiphospholipid syndrome (APS)** should be considered in ill-appearing patients who present with multiorgan failure and widespread thromboses often leading to gangrene. The combination of renal failure, acute respiratory distress syn-

drome, and cutaneous infarctions should raise the possibility of catastrophic APS (34,35).

24. If a female patient develops spontaneous skin bruising a few days after receiving a blood transfusion, order a platelet count in order to rule out **posttransfusion purpura**. Severe thrombocytopenia in this condition is caused by antibodies directed against a specific antigen on the platelets as well as antigen-free platelets (36).

25. Solid organ transplant recipients at risk for **posttransplant lymphoproliferative disorders (PTLD)** are those who have been treated with cyclosporine and azathioprine, OKT3, or high dose FK506. Pulmonary and cardiac transplantation have the highest risk of PTLD, but any solid organ transplant recipient is at risk. Epstein-Barr virus (EBV) is thought to be an integral part of the pathogenesis of this disease and those recipients who are EBV negative and receive a solid organ from an EBV-positive donor are at greatest risk of acquiring PTLD. The first step in treatment is reduction of the dosages of the immunosuppressives. The B-cell non-Hodgkin lymphoma characteristically affects extranodal sites, with unique tropism for the transplanted organ (37).

26. Fever, dyspnea, pulmonary infiltrates, weight gain, and hypotension in a patient with underlying acute promyelocytic leukemia being treated with all trans retinoic acid should raise suspicion for the **retinoic acid syndrome (RAS)**. Before attributing these symptoms to RAS, infectious causes should be ruled out (38).

27. A patient who presents with complaints of pruritus after showering should have a screening hematocrit drawn because of the possibility of **polycythemia vera** (39).

28. **Multicentric Castleman disease (MCD)** is a lymphoproliferative disorder associated with human herpesvirus 8 (HHV-8) infection. Features include fever, weight loss, generalized lymphadenopathy, and hepatosplenomegaly. Patients infected with the human immunodeficiency virus (HIV) are at increased risk

for MCD. At times, HHV-8—associated Kaposi sarcoma may simultaneously be present with MCD (40).

29. Patients with underlying **amyloidosis** may develop a bleeding diathesis secondary to the amyloid fibrils binding to specific clotting proteins (41,42).

30. A number of important **side effects** to **unfractionated heparin** therapy occur: bleeding, osteoporosis, hyperkalemia, and heparin-induced thrombocytopenia, which can lead to life-threatening venous or, less commonly, arterial thrombosis (43).

31. A patient with no underlying hematologic, oncologic (sickle cell disease, CLL) or immunosuppressive disease (acquired immunodeficiency syndrome) who presents with a profound isolated anemia with virtually absent reticulocyte response should undergo a thoracic CT scan to rule out the presence of a **thymoma**. Thymomas with or without myasthenia gravis are associated with pure red cell aplasia. The clue to the diagnosis is finding a decreased reticulocyte count. Confirmation is by bone marrow trephination demonstrating decreased or absent red blood cell progenitors. Other causes of pure red cell aplasia are idiopathic, parvovirus B19, chronic leukemia, HIV, and drug-induced anemia (44,45).

32. Bleeding that occurs in patients with **platelet disorders** differs from the type of bleeding found in patients with **factor deficiencies**. The former have mucosal bleeding (i.e., bleeding from gingiva, epistaxis, menorrhagia, and petechiae or purpura). Factor deficiency presents as bleeding into deeper tissues (e.g., hemarthrosis—bleeding into joint), bleeding into muscle, and delayed bleeding (46).

33. **Secondary hemochromatosis** should be suspected in a patient with underlying hemolytic anemia requiring frequent transfusions who presents with bronzed skin, new-onset diabetes mellitus, liver disease, and heart failure (47).

34. Two cancers that have a **low leukocyte alkaline phosphatase (LAP)** are CML and paroxysmal noc-

turnal hemoglobinuria. Occasionally, myelodysplastic syndrome can present with an LAP level of 0 (48–50).

35. **Basophilia** is an unusual hematologic abnormality and when persistent suggests leukemia, in particular CML (51).

36. The diagnosis of **idiopathic thrombocytopenic purpura (ITP)** in a patient who presents with isolated thrombocytopenia requires an HIV test, antinuclear antibody serology, and (in patients >60 years of age), a bone marrow biopsy to rule out secondary causes of ITP, which can include HIV, systemic lupus erythematosus, and myelodysplastic syndrome (52).

37. In a patient with underlying CLL, a sudden decline secondary to fevers, bulky lymphadenopathy, and abdominal pain should raise suspicion for a **Richter transformation**, which is the conversion of well-differentiated B-cell lymphocytic leukemia to a diffuse large cell lymphoma. Richter syndrome heralds a poor prognosis (53,54).

38. **Cyclic neutropenia** is defined by paroxysms of neutropenia, classically every 21 days. These episodes can be completely asymptomatic or punctuated by fevers, aphthous stomatitis, self-limited cutaneous infections, or life-threatening bacteremias from organisms such as *Clostridium septicum* (55).

REFERENCES

1. Tefferi A, Solberg LA, Silverstein MN. A clinical update in polycythemia vera and essential thrombocythemia. *Am J Med* 2000;109:141–149.
2. Poll LW, Koch JA, Vom DS, et al. Gaucher's disease of the spleen: CT and MR findings. *Abdom Imaging* 2000;25: 286–289.
3. Haran MZ, Feldberg E, Miller G, et al. Sarcoidosis presenting as massive splenomegaly and bicytopenia [Letter]. *Am J Hematol* 2000;63:232–233.
4. Bedu-Addo G, Sheldon J, Bates I. Massive splenomegaly in tropical West Africa. *Postgrad Med J* 2000;76:107–109.
5. Swaroop J, O'Reilly RA. Splenomegaly at a university hospital compared to a nearby county hospital in 317 patients. *Acta Haematol* 1999;102:83–88.

6. Fordice J, Katras T, Jackson RE, et al. Massive splenomegaly in sarcoidosis. *South Med J* 1992;85:775–778.

7. Tallman MS, Hakimian D, Peterson L. Massive splenomegaly in hairy cell leukemia. *J Clin Oncol* 1998;16:1232–1233.

8. Zuckerman E, Rosner I, Yeshurun D. Massive splenomegaly: a manifestation of active systemic lupus erythematosus [Letter]. *Clin Exp Rheumatol* 1993;11:698–699.

9. Karnam U, Rogers A. Systemic mastocytosis. *Dig Dis* 1999; 17:299–307.

10. Brain MC. Microangiopathic hemolytic anemia. *Annu Rev Med* 1970;21:133–144.

11. Brain MC. Microangiopathic hemolytic anemia. *N Engl J Med* 1969;281:833–835.

12. Nelson RL, Davis FG, Persky V, et al. Risk of neoplastic and other diseases among people with heterozygosity for hereditary hemochromatosis. *Cancer* 1995;76:875–879.

13. Biland L, Duckert F, Prisender S, et al. Quantitative estimation of coagulation factors in liver disease. The diagnostic and prognostic value of factor XIII, factor V and plasminogen. *Thromb Haemost* 1978;39:646–656.

14. Tefferi A. Myelofibrosis with myeloid metaplasia. *N Engl J Med* 2000;342:1255–1265.

15. Ramos-Casals M, Trejo O, Garcia-Carrasco M, et al. Mixed cryoglobulinemia: new concepts. *Lupus* 2000;9:83–91.

16. Robinson N, Sullivan KM. Complications of allogeneic bone marrow transplantation. *Curr Opin Hematol* 1994;1:406–411.

17. D'Souza S, Lindberg M. Typhlitis as a presenting manifestation of acute myelogenous leukemia. *South Med J* 2000;93: 218–220.

18. Schey S. Osteosclerotic myeloma and 'POEMS' syndrome. *Blood Rev* 1996;10:75–80.

19. Ebo DG, Stevens WJ. Hereditary angioneurotic edema: review of the literature. *Acta Clin Belg* 2000;55:22–29.

20. Misbah SA, Chapel HM. Adverse effects of intravenous immunoglobulin. *Drug Saf* 1993;9:254–262.

21. Jurado RL, del Rio C, Nassar G, et al. Low anion gap. *South Med J* 1998;91:624–629.

22. Renal insufficiency and failure associated with immune globulin intravenous therapy—United States, 1985–1998. *MMWR* 1999;48:518–521.

23. Hillmen P, Lewis SM, Bessler M, et al. Natural history of paroxysmal nocturnal hemoglobinuria. *N Engl J Med* 1995;333: 1253–1258.

24. Nakajima N. The change in concept and surgical treatment on Buerger's disease—personal experience and review. *Int J Cardiol* 1998;66[Suppl. 1]:S273–280; discussion S281.

25. Aqel MB, Olin JW. Thromboangiitis obliterans (Buerger's disease). *Vasc Med* 1997;2:61–66.

26. Bell WR, Starksen NF, Tong S, et al. Trousseau's syndrome. Devastating coagulopathy in the absence of heparin. *Am J Med* 1985;79:423–430.

27. Walsh-McMonagle D, Green D. Low-molecular-weight heparin in the management of Trousseau's syndrome. *Cancer* 1997;80:649–655.

28. Letai A, Kuter DJ. Cancer, coagulation, and anticoagulation. *Oncologist* 1999;4:443–449.

29. Tallman MS, Hakimian D, Kwaan HC, et al. New insights into the pathogenesis of coagulation dysfunction in acute promyelocytic leukemia. *Leuk Lymphoma* 1993;11:27–36.

30. Saper CB, Jarowski CJ. Leukemic infiltration of the cerebellum in acute myelomonocytic leukemia. *Neurology* 1992;32:77–80.

31. Myones BL, McCurdy D. The antiphospholipid syndrome: immunologic and clinical aspects. Clinical spectrum and treatment. *J Rheumatol* 2000;27[Suppl. 58]:20–28.

32. Seymour RA, Ellis JS, Thomason JM. Drug-induced gingival overgrowth and its management. *J R Coll Surg Edinb* 1993; 38:328–332.

33. Genc A, Atalay T, Gedikoglu G, et al. Leukemic children: clinical and histopathological gingival lesions. *J Clin Pediatr Dent* 1998;22:253–256.

34. Rojas-Rodriguez J, Garcia-Carrasco M, Ramos-Casals M, et al. Catastrophic antiphospholipid syndrome: clinical description and triggering factors in 8 patients. *J Rheumatol* 2000;27: 238–240.

35. Asherson RA. The catastrophic antiphospholipid syndrome, 1998. A review of the clinical features, possible pathogenesis and treatment. *Lupus* 1998;7[Suppl. 2]:S55–S62.

36. Waters AH. Post-transfusion purpura. *Blood Rev* 1989;3: 83–87.

37. Nalesnik MA. Clinicopathologic features of posttransplant lymphoproliferative disorders. *Ann Transplant* 1997;2:33–40.

38. Fenaux P, De Botton S. Retinoic acid syndrome. Recognition, prevention and management. *Drug Saf* 1998;18:273–279.

39. Fjellner B, Hagermark O. Pruritus in polycythemia vera: treatment with aspirin and possibility of platelet involvement. *Acta Derm Venereol* 1979;59:505–512.

40. Palestro G, Turrini F, Pagano M, et al. Castleman's disease. *Adv Clin Path* 1999;3:11–22.

41. Mumford AD, O'Donnell J, Gillmore JD, et al. Bleeding symptoms and coagulation abnormalities in 337 patients with AL—amyloidosis. *Br J Haematol* 2000;110:454–460.

42. Gamba G, Montani N, Anesi E, et al. Clotting alterations in primary systemic amyloidosis. *Haematologica* 2000;85:289–292.

43. Bick RL, Frenkel EP. Clinical aspects of heparin-induced thrombocytopenia and thrombosis and other side effects of heparin therapy. *Clin Appl Thromb Hemost* 1999;5[Suppl. 1]: S7–S15.

44. Mamiya S, Itoh T, Miura AB. Acquired pure red cell aplasia in Japan. *Eur J Haematol* 1997;59:199–205.

45. Thomas CR, Wright CD, Loehrer PJ. Thymoma: state of the art. *J Clin Oncol* 1999;17:2280–2289.

46. McCrae K. Approach to the patient with bleeding. In: Humes HD, ed. *Kelley's textbook of internal medicine*. Philadelphia: Lippincott Williams & Wilkins, 2000:1606–1613.

47. Schafer AI, Cheron RG, Dluhy R, et al. Clinical consequences of acquired transfusional iron overload in adults. *N Engl J Med* 1981;304:319–324.

48. DePalma L, Delgado P, Werner M. Diagnostic discrimination and cost effective assay strategy for leukocyte alkaline phosphatase. *Clin Chim Acta* 1996;244:83–90.

49. Rambaldi A, Terao M, Bettoni S, et al. Differences in the expression of alkaline phosphatase mRNA in chronic myelogenous leukemia and paroxysmal nocturnal hemoglobinuria polymorphonuclear leukocytes. *Blood* 1989;73:1113–1115.

50. Okamoto T, Okada M, Yamada S, et al. Flow-cytometric analysis of leukocyte alkaline phosphatase in myelodysplastic syndromes. *Acta Haematol* 1999;102:89–93.

51. Arnalich F, Lahoz C, Larrocha C, et al. Incidence and clinical significance of peripheral and bone marrow basophilia. *J Med* 1987;18:293–303.

52. Chong BH, Keng TB. Advances in the diagnosis of idiopathic thrombocytopenic purpura. *Semin Hematol* 2000;37:249–260.

53. Giles FJ, O'Brien SM, Keating MJ. Chronic lymphocytic leukemia in (Richter's) transformation. *Semin Oncol* 1998;25: 117–125.

54. Long JC, Aisenberg AC. Richter's syndrome. A terminal complication of chronic lymphocytic leukemia with distinct clinicopathologic features. *Am J Clin Pathol* 1975;63:786–795.

55. Dale DC, Hammond WP. Cyclic neutropenia: a clinical review. *Blood Rev* 1988;2:178–185.

7

INFECTIOUS DISEASES

1. The **Eagle effect** states that as group A streptococci (GAS) inoculum divides in a logarithmic phase, their penicillin-binding proteins become down regulated. Cell wall active agents such as penicillin may be less effective. This is one of the reasons high-dose clindamycin therapy is added to penicillin to treat serious necrotizing infections with GAS or *Clostridium perfringens* gas gangrene. Clindamycin is able to disrupt protein synthesis and, theoretically, block toxin production (1).

2. **Aztreonam** does not cause anaphylaxis in patients with documented penicillin-induced anaphylaxis (2,3).

3. **Myasthenia gravis** is a contraindication to aminoglycoside use because of the potential for increased neuromuscular blockade. Other agents that should be avoided include β-blockers, quinine, quinidine, succinylcholine, and phenytoin (4,5).

4. **Aminoglycoside vestibular toxicity** usually causes difficulty maintaining balance, especially in the dark, and oscillopsia, a condition where objects appear to be moving back and forth while the head of the patient is moving. True vertigo is a less common manifestation because it involves acute, bilateral vestibular loss and, thus, no asymmetry in function (6).

5. Once-a-day dosing of an aminoglycoside is possible because of its **post-antibiotic effect (PAE)** and **concentration-dependent killing (CDK)**. PAE refers to continued suppression of bacterial growth beyond the effective $T^{1/2}$ of the drug. Antibiotics that demonstrate CDK have a greater bactericidal effect at higher peak concentrations (7).

6. The anti-mycobacterial medication rifabutin is an important cause of **drug-induced anterior uveitis**, especially in immunodeficient patients. It is usually reversible when therapy is discontinued (8).

7. Stroke in a young person, especially when accompanied by fever, is **endocarditis** until proved otherwise (9,10).

8. Some organisms to consider in **culture negative endocarditis** are the HACEK group (*Haemophilus aphrophilus, H. parainfluenzae, Actinobacillus actinomycetemcomitans, Cardiobacterium hominis, Eikenella corrodens,* and *Kingella kingae*), *Bartonella henselae, Coxiella burnetii, Brucella* sp., *Tropheryma whippelii, Aspergillus, Mycoplasma pneumoniae,* and *Chlamydia psittaci.* Some of these fastidious organisms require up to 2 weeks of growth in culture. Ask the microbiology laboratory to consider these organisms and not to discard the cultures prematurely (11).

9. Gentamicin, which acts synergistically with cell-wall active antibiotics (oxacillin, nafcillin) in the treatment of **enterococcal endocarditis,** has been shown to clear bacteremia more rapidly in patients with *Staphylococcus aureus* **endocarditis**. This effect, however, does not change clinical outcome (12).

10. Vancomycin is inferior to nafcillin for the treatment of **methicillin-sensitive *S. aureus* endocarditis** (13).

11. A **splenic infarct** should heighten suspicion for infective endocarditis (14).

12. In the workup of **fever of unknown origin (FUO)**, remember the longer the duration of fever, the less likely the diagnosis is to be infectious [fevers that last greater than 6 months are rarely infectious (6%)] (15).

13. **Fever** in a patient who has **traveled** outside the United States suggests three initial diagnoses: malaria, typhoid fever, and dengue (16).

14. The finding of **bilateral adrenal enlargement** in a patient with FUO can be a clue to underlying tuberculosis or histoplasmosis (17,18).

15. **Drug fever** should abate by 48 hours after discontinuing the offending agent. If fevers continue after this time, continue to search for an underlying cause (19).

16. Patients who present with recurrent *Neisseria meningitidis* infections should be tested for **terminal complement deficiency** (20).

17. The **splenectomized** patient who is bitten by a dog and becomes febrile and hypotensive likely is septic from the bacterium *Capnocytophaga canimorsus*, formerly known as "dysgonic fermenter 2" (DF-2) (21,22).

18. **Strongyloides hyperinfection syndrome** should be considered in an immunocompromised patient who presents with eosinophilia, generalized abdominal pain, pulmonary infiltrates, and gram-negative bacteremia. Hyperinfection can occur with overwhelming larval penetration into the lungs and other tissues (23,24).

19. Giardiasis should be suspected in a patient with underlying **common variable immunodeficiency disease** who presents with chronic diarrhea. These patients have a substantially increased risk of infection with the parasite *Giardia lamblia*, which, in part, may be due to decreased secretory IgA (25).

20. The mortality rate of a patient with **neutropenic fever** who has an organism identified by blood culture is approximately 25%. Fortunately, organisms are identified in the minority of cases (26).

21. In a patient with a previous splenectomy, pneumococcus is the leading organism involved in **overwhelming post-splenectomized sepsis (OPSS)**. Hypoglycemia is a clue to OPSS caused by pneumococcus (27–29).

22. Bacillus Calmette-Guérin (BCG) vaccination is a live attenuated form of *Mycobacterium bovis* and should not be given to immunocompromised hosts for fear of precipitating **disseminated BCGosis** (30).

23. **Actinomycosis** should be suspected in a patient who develops pelvic inflammatory disease in the setting of an intrauterine contraceptive device (31).

24. The finding of candidemia should prompt an ophthalmologic evaluation to rule out **candidal endophthalmitis**, which can lead to permanent blindness if not treated early and aggressively (32).

25. Septic thrombophlebitis of the jugular vein is called **Lemierre syndrome** and the causative agent is *Fusobacterium necrophorum*. It is a "paramandibular space infection" involving the posterior compartment of the lateral pharyngeal space. Typically, it presents with tenderness at the angle of the jaw, but little or nothing is actually seen short of a computed tomography (CT) scan. The emboli typically go to the joints and lung according to the 20 cases described by Lemierre in 1936 (33,34).

26. Most **subdural empyemas** are secondary to local extension from sinusitis, whereas otitis media and mastoiditis are relatively less common causes (35).

27. A patient who presents with fever and back pain, along with focal spinous process tenderness on palpation, should be considered to have an **epidural abscess** until proved otherwise. Fever, which is a helpful clue, is not present in mechanical causes of back pain. Magnetic resonance imaging (MRI) is a sensitive imaging modality for the early diagnosis of epidural abscess. It is imperative to think of this diagnosis before neurologic deterioration (extremity weakness, bowel or bladder incontinence, paralysis) occurs because the earlier the institution of surgical drainage and antibiotic therapy, the greater the chance of preserving neurologic function (36).

28. The differential diagnosis of infections that cause **persistent chronic meningitis** are *Cryptococcal neoformans*, *Treponema pallidum*, *M. tuberculosis*, *Borrelia burgdorferi* (agent of Lyme disease), *B. henselae* (agent of cat-scratch disease), and endemic mycoses (*Histoplasmosis capsulatum* and *Coccidioides immitis*). It should be noted that few patients survive longer than 4 to 6 weeks with untreated tuberculous meningitis (37).

29. Three important causes of severe **hyperthermia** are heat stroke, neuroleptic malignant syndrome, and malignant hyperthermia. The history is vital, especially because the clinical manifestations of all three are protean, including rigidity, delirium, seizures, disseminated intravascular coagulation, myocardial infarction, acute respiratory distress syndrome (ARDS), rhabdomyolysis, renal failure, electrolyte disturbances, autonomic dysfunction, labile blood pressure, and arrhythmias. Remember, infectious diseases rarely cause temperatures greater than 41°C (38).

30. An influenzalike illness that rapidly progresses to severe hypoxemia, in addition to a widened mediastinum on chest x-ray study, suggests a diagnosis of **inhalational anthrax**, which has a treated 80% mortality. If bacillus is cultured in this setting, it is important not to allow the laboratory to discard the organism as a contaminant, but rather ascertain speciation to identify B. anthracis. Anthrax is one of the more feared organisms used for biological warfare (39).

31. Large cystic masses seen on the CT scan of the chest in a patient from an area endemic with sheep may be secondary to the cestode *Echinococcal granulosus* leading to **pulmonary hydatid disease**. One diagnostic test is serology for echinococcal IgG antibodies. Most patients with echinococcal pulmonary cysts do not have liver involvement, although they can occur concurrently (40).

32. **Acute rheumatic fever**, a nonsuppurative sequelae of group A streptococcal pharyngitis, has virtually disappeared in developed countries. It is not seen with poststreptococcal cellulitis or impetigo (41).

33. The most common cause of **generalized lymphadenopathy** in the outpatient setting is Epstein-Barr virus assuming the form of infectious mononucleosis. The broader differential diagnosis of generalized superficial adenopathy includes infections (human immunodeficiency virus, cytomegalovirus, syphilis, toxoplasmosis), malignancies (lymphoma), rheuma-

tologic disease (systemic lupus erythematous), miscellaneous diseases (Castleman disease and sarcoidosis), and phenytoin hypersensitivity (42).

34. A few infectious diseases cause **pulse-temperature dissociation**: *Salmonella typhi*, *C. burnetii* (agent of Q fever), *Chlamydia* sp., and dengue fever. Any intracellular organism has the potential to cause a relative bradycardia (Faget sign) (43–45).

35. There is little benefit to culturing a wound in a patient with underlying diabetes and vascular insufficiency who presents with a **nonhealing ulcer** in a distal extremity. The organisms (classically polymicrobial) responsible can be identified through bone biopsy or blood cultures (46).

36. The yield of sending stool cultures for routine bacteria, ova, and parasites in an immunocompetent patient who experiences diarrhea initially on day 3 of hospitalization is too insignificant to be helpful. *Clostridium difficile* is the leading infectious cause of nosocomial diarrhea and is the only organism that should be considered in the workup of nosocomial diarrhea in an immunocompetent patient. The other major cause of hospital-acquired diarrhea is medication side effects (47).

37. **Enterohemorrhagic *Escherichia coli*** (EHEC) colitis usually presents with severe abdominal pain and bloody stools. Fever is oftentimes absent. Many experts feel EHEC should not be treated with antibiotics because of the increased incidence of hemolytic-uremic syndrome, although data are conflicting. Patients who present with bloody diarrhea should have their stools examined for *E. coli* O157:H7, especially young children and the elderly (48,49).

38. Frontal sinusitis, headache, fever, and swelling of the forehead, suggest the possibility of **frontal bone osteomyelitis** (Potts puffy tumor) (50).

39. The most common location for **vertebral osteomyelitis** depends on both the organism and the host. Intravenous drug users are predisposed to pseudo-

monal osteomyelitis of the spine, whereas patients with urinary catheters in place for long periods tend to suffer from lumbar vertebral osteomyelitis (51).

40. *S. aureus* is the most common organism implicated in **osteomyelitis**. However, in young patients with underlying sickle cell anemia and osteomyelitis, *Salmonella* organisms may be responsible (52).

41. A patient who presents with the abrupt onset of fevers, severe headache, myalgias, and dry cough, with a chest x-ray study consistent with pneumonia and no improvement on β-lactam antibiotics may be infected with an atypical organism (mycoplasma, *C. pneumoniae*, or legionella). If the patient has had exposure to birds, in particular parrots, also consider **C. psittaci**. Extrapulmonary manifestations of psittacosis include splenomegaly, erythema nodosum, horder spots (erythematous macules on the trunk), hepatitis, and culture negative endocarditis (53,54).

42. **Friedlander bacillus** is an eponym for *Klebsiella pneumoniae*, the agent responsible for community-acquired pneumonia in alcoholic men greater than 40 years of age who produce a sputum that looks like "currant jelly." This pneumonia can mimic pneumococcal pneumonia, but differs in that it more often results in pulmonary abscesses (55).

43. **Candida pneumonia** is exceedingly uncommon. The small nodules seen on chest x-ray study are a reflection of candidemia. Candida is almost never acquired through a respiratory route (56).

44. *Serratia marcescens* pneumonia should be considered in a patient who presents with shortness of breath, pulmonary infiltrates, and **heme-negative "hemoptysis."** Some strains of the organism produce a pigment that colors the sputum red (57).

45. **Hantavirus pulmonary syndrome** should be considered in an otherwise healthy adult from an endemic area who presents in ARDS and hypotension with exposure to rodents within the past 4 weeks (58).

46. A patient with **hemochromatosis** who presents in extremis with fever and hypotension may have bacterial sepsis with either *Yersinia enterocolitica* or *Vibrio vulnificus*, two organisms that thrive in iron-rich media (59,60).

47. Consider the late complications of **typhoid fever** that can occur around the third or fourth week of illness (e.g., intestinal perforation and necrotizing cholecystitis) (61).

48. A young, healthy woman who presents with unexplained hypotension may have **staphylococcal toxic shock syndrome**. Other features of this syndrome include fevers, headache, confusion, abdominal pain, and diarrhea. Elevated aminotransferases and renal insufficiency are also common. This can occur during menstruation in women who use highly absorbent tampons. In this syndrome, *S. aureus* is usually not cultured from the blood in contrast to streptococcal toxic shock syndrome. The diagnosis can be made via vaginal cultures (62,63).

49. **Hemorrhagic bullae** in an ill patient with underlying cirrhosis should raise the specter of bacteremia secondary to *Vibrio vulnificus*. This comma-shaped, gram-negative rod can be acquired by eating raw shellfish and has a high mortality rate in patients with underlying liver disease (64,65).

50. ***Propionibacterium acnes*** is an anaerobic, gram-positive rod that is a frequent contaminant of cultures, but is an important pathogen in shunt-related infections. This is one of the uncommon anaerobes resistant to metronidazole (66,67).

51. Shock associated with ***S. typhi*** bacteremia is treated with antibiotics in addition to corticosteroids. Addition of steroids to antibiotics has been shown to improve survival in typhoidal sepsis (68).

52. Documentation of *Streptococcus sanguis* or *S. mutans* bacteremia should prompt a search for **endocarditis** (69,70).

53. A patient who becomes febrile, hypotensive, and develops a rash 1–6 hours after antibiotic treatment for primary or secondary syphilis likely has the **Jarisch-Herxheimer reaction**. This represents the destruction of spirochetes by antibiotics with the release of treponemal antigens into the bloodstream. It is usually a self-limited reaction and can be prevented by pretreatment with tumor necrosis factor-α (TNF-α) antibodies (71).

54. Syphilis is one of the more common causes of **infectious uveitis** (72).

55. The advantage of treating **Lyme disease** with doxycycline is that coincident infection with **human granulocytic *Ehrlichiosis*** (both carried by the same deer tick) can also be treated effectively (73).

56. In patients who have an illness suggestive of **Lyme disease** that lasts greater than 1 month, a persistently positive IgM alone is likely to reflect a false-positive result and argues against the diagnosis of Lyme disease (74).

57. Meningococcemia and Rocky Mountain spotted fever (RMSF) are two potentially life-threatening diseases that can present with **fever** and **palpable purpura**. Clinical differentiation is important in order to select proper antibiotic therapy. The palpable purpura of meningococcemia appears soon after symptoms of upper respiratory tract infection, fever, and meningitis, whereas the palpable purpura of RMSF is typically preceded by several days of fevers, chills, and severe headache. The initial erythematous macules or papules of RMSF typically begin on the ankles, wrists, palms or soles, and then spread centripetally to involve the trunk before becoming purpuric (75–77).

58. Lyme disease can cause a wide array of symptoms; however, none of these should cause a patient to appear very sick. In the presence of Lyme disease and an ill-appearing patient, consider two other infections that can be acquired by the bite of the same tick that harbors the lyme spirochete, namely the para-

site **Babesia microti** and the rickettsia **Ehrlichia chaffeensis**. Babesiosis, also known as Nantucket fever, can cause shaking chills, high fevers, and a pronounced hemolytic anemia (similar to malaria), whereas ehrlichiosis causes leukopenia, severe headache, increased aminotransferases, thrombocytopenia, and fevers. Case reports have been made of simultaneous transmission of all three organisms by the *Ixodes* tick. Lyme disease, alone, should not cause high fevers (78,79).

59. Systemic glucocorticoids should be used as adjunctive therapy to antibiotics in patients with **tuberculous pericarditis** (survival benefit). Whereas, the benefit of glucocorticoids in adults with tuberculous meningitis is less clear (80,81).

60. **Tuberculous spondylitis** (Pott disease) classically targets the lower thoracic and upper lumbar spine (60,82,83).

61. A patient with underlying pyelonephritis who fails to defervesce after 3 days of antibiotics should have an imaging study of the kidneys to rule out the presence of a **perinephric abscess** (84).

62. Recurrent urinary tract infections (UTI) and a urine pH consistently documented between 7 and 9 should raise suspicion of gram-negative **urease-producing bacteria** (e.g., *Proteus mirabilis*, or less commonly *Klebsiella*, *Pseudomonas*, and *Ureaplasma*). These urease-producing organisms can raise the urinary ammonium concentrations, creating struvite stones (magnesium ammonium phosphate) which can become secondarily infected, serving as a nidus for recurrent UTI (85–87).

63. A UTI in a man greater than 40 years of age is **prostatitis** until proved otherwise. Middle-aged men do not commonly have isolated acute cystitis (88).

64. **Staphylococcal** organisms in the urine should prompt an investigation for staphylococcal bacteremia and endocarditis, in the absence of an indwelling Foley catheter (89,90).

65. **Asymptomatic bacteriuria** (a positive urine culture without symptoms of UTI or pyuria) should only be treated in a small number of clinical settings: pregnancy, patients awaiting urologic procedures, patients who have a bladder catheter, children with vesicoureteral reflux, and patients with struvite stones (surgery first-line treatment) (91).

66. Herpes zoster on the tip of the nose implies that the nasociliary branch of the ophthalmic nerve (V1) is affected, suggesting a greater risk for ophthalmic involvement with zoster. A zoster vesicle at the tip of the nose is **Hutchinson sign** (92).

67. **Herpes simplex type I encephalitis** is an important diagnosis to consider in any patient with fever, mental status changes, personality changes, or seizures. A lumbar puncture (LP) typically shows a monocytic pleocytosis in addition to elevated protein and red blood cells. An LP without pleocytosis should prompt a search for other causes of encephalopathy. Herpes virus can be demonstrated in the cerebrospinal fluid by polymerase chain reaction. A negative result essentially rules out the diagnosis of herpes simplex virus type I encephalitis. MRI may demonstrate temporal lobe changes as early as 2–3 days from the onset of symptoms. Early antiviral treatment is essential to prevent permanent neurologic sequelae (93,94).

68. Patients who present with **fulminant hepatitis B virus (HBV)** infection may have cleared their HbsAg before seeking medical attention. In these rare cases of HBsAg-negative fulminant hepatic failure, ordering HBV DNA or IgM antiHBc may confirm the diagnosis (95).

69. Rarely, patients with zoster ophthalmicus will go on to have a contralateral hemiplegia, which is secondary to a **zoster-associated vasculitis** (96).

70. The combination of polyarthritis and urticaria should point toward a diagnosis of **HBV infection**, causing an immune complex-mediated disease. The arthralgias and arthritis are usually sudden, additive, and

symmetric, affecting the knees and hands most commonly, although any joint can be affected. Hepatitis A and C can cause similar features, although not as commonly as HBV. It should be noted that the arthritis often occurs before jaundice develops (97).

71. Of the **aminoglycosides**, tobramycin typically has the lowest minimum inhibitory concentration against pseudomonas (most potent). Amikacin is usually the aminoglycoside that harbors the least resistance among aminoglycoside-resistant bacilli (98,99).

72. Antibiotic sensitivity panels to gram-negative rods that show sensitivity to a second generation cephalosporin, but resistance to a third generation cephalosporin, warrant further investigation. Some of these gram-negative rods (e.g., *E. coli* or *K. pneumoniae*) may have **extended spectrum β-lactamase**, which makes them resistant to the cephalosporins as a group (100).

REFERENCES

1. Stevens DL, Gibbons AE, Bergstrom R, et al. The Eagle effect revisited: efficacy of clindamycin, erythromycin, and penicillin in the treatment of streptococcal myositis. *J Infect Dis* 1988;158:23–28.
2. Saxon A, Hassner A, Swabb EA, et al. Lack of cross-reactivity between aztreonam, a monobactam antibiotic, and penicillin in penicillin-allergic subjects. *J Infect Dis* 1984;149:16–22.
3. Loria RC, Finnerty N, Wedner HJ. Successful use of aztreonam in a patient who failed oral penicillin desensitization. *J Allergy Clin Immunol* 1989;83:735–737.
4. Hokkanen E, Toivakka E. Streptomycin-induced neuromuscular fatigue in myasthenia gravis. *Ann Clin Res* 1969;1: 220–226.
5. Kaeser HE. Drug-induced myasthenic syndromes. *Acta Neurol Scand Suppl* 1984;100:39–47.
6. Ramsden RT, Ackrill P. Bobbing oscillopsia from gentamicin toxicity. *Br J Audiol* 1982;16:147–150.
7. Preston SL, Briceland LL. Single daily dosing of aminoglycosides. *Pharmacotherapy* 1995;15:297–316.
8. Becker K, Schimkat M, Jablonowski H, et al. Anterior uveitis associated with rifabutin medication in AIDS patients. *Infection* 1996;24:34–36.

9. Case records of the Massachusetts General Hospital. Weekly clinicopathological exercises. Case 10-1993. A 67-year-old man with mitral regurgitation and an abrupt onset of ataxia and fever. *N Engl J Med* 1993;328:717–725.

10. Salgado AV, Furlan AJ, Keys TF, et al. Neurologic complications of endocarditis: a 12-year experience. *Neurology* 1989;39:173–178.

11. Berbari EF, Cockerill FR 3, Steckelberg JM. Infective endocarditis due to unusual or fastidious microorganisms. *Mayo Clin Proc* 1997;72:532–542.

12. Sande MA, Courtney KB. Nafcillin-gentamicin synergism in experimental staphylococcal endocarditis. *J Lab Clin Med* 1976;88:118–124.

13. Small PM, Chambers HF. Vancomycin for Staphylococcus aureus endocarditis in intravenous drug users. *Antimicrob Agents Chemother* 1990;34:1227–1231.

14. Ting W, Silverman NA, Arzouman DA, et al. Splenic septic emboli in endocarditis. *Circulation* 1990;82:IV105–IV109.

15. Gelfand JR, Dinarello CA. Fever of unknown origin. In: Fauci AS, Braunwald E, Isselbacher KJ, et al., eds. *Harrison's principles of internal medicine*, Vol. 1. New York: McGraw-Hill, 1998:780–785.

16. Suh KN, Kozarsky PE, Keystone JS. Evaluation of fever in the returned traveler. *Med Clin North Am* 1999;83:997–1017.

17. Giacaglia LR, Lin CJ, Lucon AM, et al. Disseminated histoplasmosis presenting as bilateral adrenal masses. *Rev Hosp Clin Fac Med Sao Paulo* 1998;53:254–256.

18. Wang YX, Chen CR, He GX, et al. CT findings of adrenal glands in patients with tuberculous Addison's disease. *J Belge Radiol* 1998;81:226–228.

19. Lipsky BA, Hirschmann JV. Drug fever. *JAMA* 1981;245:851–854.

20. Wurzner R, Orren A, Lachmann PJ. Inherited deficiencies of the terminal components of human complement. *Immunodefic Rev* 1992;3:123–147.

21. Ruddock TL, Rindler JM, Bergfeld WF. Capnocytophaga canimorsus septicemia in an asplenic patient. *Cutis* 1997;60:95–97.

22. Vanhonsebrouck AY, Gordts B, Wauters G, et al. Fatal septicemia with Capnocytophaga canimorsus in a compromised host. A case report with review of the literature. *Acta Clin Belg* 1991;46:364–370.

23. Casati A, Cornero G, Muttini S, et al. Hyperacute pneumonitis in a patient with overwhelming Strongyloides stercoralis infection. *Eur J Anaesthesiol* 1996;13:498–501.

24. Bradley SL, Dines DE, Brewer NS. Disseminated Strongyloides stercoralis in an immunosuppressed host. *Mayo Clin Proc* 1978;53:332–335.

25. Cunningham-Rundles C. Clinical and immunologic studies of common variable immunodeficiency. *Curr Opin Pediatr* 1994;6:676–681.

26. Gonzalez-Barca E, Fernandez-Sevilla A, Carratala J, et al. Prognostic factors influencing mortality in cancer patients with neutropenia and bacteremia. *Eur J Clin Microbiol Infect Dis* 1999;18:539–544.

27. Miller SI, Wallace RJ Jr., Musher DM, et al. Hypoglycemia as a manifestation of sepsis. *Am J Med.* 1980;68:649–654.

28. Latos DL, Stone WJ. Fulminant pneumococcal bacteremia in an asplenic chronic hemodialysis patient. *Johns Hopkins Med J* 1978;143:165–168.

29. Torres J, Bisno AL. Hyposplenism and pneumococcemia. Visualization of Diplococcus pneumoniae in the peripheral blood smear. *Am J Med* 1973;55:851–855.

30. Talbot EA, Perkins MD, Silva SF, et al. Disseminated bacille Calmette-Guerin disease after vaccination: case report and review [see comments]. *Clin Infect Dis* 1997;24:1139–1146.

31. Hager WD, Majmudar B. Pelvic actinomycosis in women using intrauterine contraceptive devices. *Am J Obstet Gynecol* 1979;133:60–63.

32. Patel BC, Kaye SB, Morgan LH. Candidal endophthalmitis: a manifestation of systemic candidiasis. *Postgrad Med J* 1987;63:563–565.

33. Goldenberg D, Golz A, Joachims HZ. Retropharyngeal abscess: a clinical review. *J Laryngol Otol* 1997;111:546–550.

34. Golpe R, Marin B, Alonso M. Lemierre's syndrome (necrobacillosis). *Postgrad Med J* 1999;75:141–144.

35. Dill SR, Cobbs CG, McDonald CK. Subdural empyema: analysis of 32 cases and review. *Clin Infect Dis* 1995;20:372–386.

36. Rigamonti D, Liem L, Sampath P, et al. Spinal epidural abscess: contemporary trends in etiology, evaluation, and management. *Surg Neurol* 1999;52:189–196; discussion 197.

37. Koroshetz WJ, Swartz MN. Chronic and recurrent meningitis. In: Fauci AS, Braunwald E, Isselbacher KJ, et al., eds. *Harrison's principles of internal medicine.* New York: McGraw-Hill, 1998:2434–2439.

38. Denborough M. Malignant hyperthermia [see comments]. *Lancet* 1998;352:1131–1136.

39. Dixon TC, Meselson M, Guillemin J, et al. Anthrax. *N Engl J Med* 1999;341:815–826.

40. Bhatia G. Echinococcus. *Semin Respir Infect* 1997;12:171–186.

41. Kaplan EL, Anthony BF, Chapman SS, et al. The influence of the site of infection on the immune response to group A streptococci. *J Clin Invest* 1970;49:1405–1414.

42. Ferrer R. Lymphadenopathy: differential diagnosis and evaluation [see comments]. *Am Fam Physician* 1998;58: 1313–1320.

43. Cunha BA, Quintiliani R. The atypical pneumonias: a diagnostic and therapeutic approach. *Postgrad Med* 1979;66: 95–102.

44. Gubler DJ. Dengue and dengue hemorrhagic fever. *Clin Microbiol Rev* 1998;11:480–496.

45. Ostergaard L, Huniche B, Andersen PL. Relative bradycardia in infectious diseases. *J Infect* 1996;33:185–191.

46. Gerding DN. Foot infections in diabetic patients: the role of anaerobes. *Clin Infect Dis* 1995;20[Suppl. 2]:S283–S288.

47. Cunha BA. Nosocomial diarrhea. *Crit Care Clin* 1998;14: 329–338.

48. Cohen MB, Giannella RA. Hemorrhagic colitis associated with *Escherichia coli* O157:H7. *Adv Intern Med* 1992;37: 173–195.

49. Wong CS, Jelacic S, Habeeb RL, et al. The risk of the hemolytic-uremic syndrome after antibiotic treatment of Escherichia coli O157:H7 infections [see comments]. *N Engl J Med* 2000;342:1930–1936.

50. Babu RP, Todor R, Kasoff SS. Pott's puffy tumor: the forgotten entity. Case report. *J Neurosurg* 1996;84:110–112.

51. Lew DP, Waldvogel FA. Osteomyelitis [see comments]. *N Engl J Med* 1997;336:999–1007.

52. Burnett MW, Bass JW, Cook BA. Etiology of osteomyelitis complicating sickle cell disease. *Pediatrics* 1998;101: 296–297.

53. Yung AP, Grayson ML. Psittacosis–a review of 135 cases. *Med J Aust* 1998;148:228–233.

54. Kirchner JT. Psittacosis. Is contact with birds causing your patient's pneumonia? *Postgrad Med* 1997;102:181–182, 187–188, 193–194.

55. Fuxench-Lopez Z, Ramirez-Ronda CH. Pharyngeal flora in ambulatory alcoholic patients: prevalence of gram-negative bacilli. *Arch Intern Med* 1978;138:1815–1816.

56. Walsh TJ, Pizzo PA. Candidiasis. In: Kassirer JP, Greene HL, III, eds. *Current therapy in adult medicine.* St. Louis: Mosby-Year Book, 1997:255.

57. Hurtado Ayuso JE, Otero Candelera R, Lopez Casanova C. Pseudo-hemoptysis due to *Serratia marcescens*, an etiology to remember [Letter]. *Arch.Bronconeumol* 1999;35:194–195.

58. Update: hantavirus pulmonary syndrome—United States, 1999. *MMWR* 1999;48:521–525.

59. Bullen JJ, Spalding PB, Ward CG, et al. Hemochromatosis, iron and septicemia caused by Vibrio vulnificus. *Arch Intern Med* 1991;151:1606–1609.

60. Abbott M, Galloway A, Cunningham JL. Haemochromatosis presenting with a double *Yersinia* infection. *J Infect* 1986; 13:143–145.

61. Keusch G. Salmonellosis. In: Fauci AS, Braunwald E, Isselbacher E, et al., eds. *Harrison's principles of internal medicine*. New York: McGraw-Hill, 1998:951–954.

62. Williams GR. The toxic shock syndrome [see comments]. *BMJ* 1990;300:960.

63. Petitti DB, Reingold A. Tampon characteristics and menstrual toxic shock syndrome [Letter]. *JAMA* 1988;259:686–687.

64. Linkous DA, Oliver JD. Pathogenesis of *Vibrio vulnificus*. *FEMS Microbiol Lett* 1999;174:207–214.

65. Vollberg CM, Herrera JL. *Vibrio vulnificus* infection: an important cause of septicemia in patients with cirrhosis. *South Med J* 1997;90:1040–1042.

66. Thompson TP, Albright AL. Propionibacterium [correction of Proprionibacterium] acnes infections of cerebrospinal fluid shunts. *Childs Nerv Syst* 1998;14:378–380.

67. Collignon PJ, Munro R, Morris G. Susceptibility of anaerobic bacteria to antimicrobial agents. *Pathology* 1988;20:48–52.

68. Thompson J. Role of glucocorticosteroids in the treatment of infectious diseases. *Eur J Clin Microbiol Infect Dis.* 1993; 12[Suppl. 1]:S68–S72.

69. Harder EJ, Wilkowske CJ, Washington JA 2d, et al. Streptococcus mutans endocarditis. *Ann Intern Med* 1974;80: 364–368.

70. Watanakunakorn C, Pantelakis J. Alpha-hemolytic streptococcal bacteremia: a review of 203 episodes during 1980–1991. *Scand J Infect Dis* 1993;25:403–408.

71. Fekade D, Knox K, Hussein K, et al. Prevention of Jarisch-Herxheimer reactions by treatment with antibodies against tumor necrosis factor alpha [see comments]. *N Engl J Med* 1996;335:311–315.

72. Dunn JP, Nozik RA. Uveitis: role of the physician in treating systemic causes. *Geriatrics* 1994;49:27–32.

73. Nadelman RB, Horowitz HW, Hsieh TC, et al. Simultaneous human granulocytic ehrlichiosis and Lyme borreliosis. *N Engl J Med* 1997;337:27–30.

74. Steere AC. Diagnosis and treatment of Lyme arthritis. *Med Clin North Am* 1997;81:179–194.

75. Drage LA. Life-threatening rashes: dermatologic signs of four infectious diseases. *Mayo Clin Proc* 1999;74:68–72.

76. Kirk JL, Fine DP, Sexton DJ, et al. Rocky Mountain spotted fever. A clinical review based on 48 confirmed cases, 1943–1986. *Medicine (Baltimore)* 1990;69:35–45.

77. Helmick CG, Bernard KW, D'Angelo LJ. Rocky Mountain spotted fever: clinical, laboratory, and epidemiological features of 262 cases. *J Infect Dis* 1984;150:480–488.

78. Dumler JS, Bakken JS. Human ehrlichioses: newly recognized infections transmitted by ticks. *Annu Rev Med* 1998; 49:201–213.

79. Pruthi RK, Marshall WF, Wiltsie JC, et al. Human babesiosis. *Mayo Clin Proc* 1995;70:853–862.

80. Strang JI. Rapid resolution of tuberculous pericardial effusions with high dose prednisone and anti-tuberculous drugs. *J Infect* 1994;28:251–254.

81. Coyle PK. Glucocorticoids in central nervous system bacterial infection. *Arch Neurol* 1999;56:796–801.

82. Case records of the Massachusetts General Hospital. Weekly clinicopathological exercises. Case 9-1996. A 21-year-old African woman with thoracolumbar pain and fever [clinical conference]. *N Engl J Med* 1996;334:784–789.

83. Reinicke V, Korner B. Fulminant septicemia caused by *Yersinia enterocolitica*. *Scand J Infect Dis* 1977;9:249–251.

84. Hutchison FN, Kaysen GA. Perinephric abscess: the missed diagnosis. *Med Clin North Am* 1988;72:993–1014.

85. McLean RJ, Downey J, Clapham L, et al. A simple technique for studying struvite crystal growth in vitro. *Urol Res* 1990;18:39–43.

86. McLean RJ, Nickel JC, Cheng KJ, et al. The ecology and pathogenicity of urease-producing bacteria in the urinary tract. *Crit Rev Microbiol* 1988;16:37–79.

87. Rothenberg ME. Eosinophilia. *N Engl J Med* 1998;338: 1592–1600.

88. Lipsky BA. Urinary tract infections in men. Epidemiology, pathophysiology, diagnosis, and treatment. *Ann Intern Med* 1989;110:138–150.

89. Deresiewicz RI, Parsonnet L. Staphylococcal Infections. In: Fauci AS, Braunwald E, Isselbacher E, et al., eds. *Harrison's principles of internal medicine*. New York: McGraw-Hill, 1998:875–885.

90. Lee BK, Crossley K, Gerding DN. The association between *Staphylococcus aureus* bacteremia and bacteriuria. *Am J Med* 1978;65:303–306.

91. O'Donnell JA, Abrutyn E. Urinary tract infection. In: Kassirer JP, Greene HL, III, eds. *Current therapy in adult medicine*. St. Louis: Mosby-Year Book, 1997:253–255.

92. Tomkinson A, Roblin DG, Brown MJ. Hutchinson's sign and its importance in rhinology. *Rhinology (Leiden)* 1995;33: 180–182.

93. Skoldenberg B. Herpes simplex encephalitis. *Scand J Infect Dis Suppl* 1991;80:40–46.

94. Domingues RB, Tsanaclis AM, Pannuti CS, et al. Evaluation of the range of clinical presentations of herpes simplex encephalitis by using polymerase chain reaction assay of cerebrospinal fluid samples. *Clin Infect Dis* 1997;25:86–91.

95. Wright TL, Mamish D, Combs C, et al. Hepatitis B virus and apparent fulminant non-A, non-B hepatitis [see comments]. *Lancet* 1992;339:952–955.

96. Reshef E, Greenberg SB, Jankovic J. Herpes zoster ophthalmicus followed by contralateral hemiparesis: report of two cases and review of literature. *J Neurol Neurosurg Psychiatry* 1985;48:122–127.

97. Pease C, Keat A. Arthritis as the main or only symptom of hepatitis B infection. *Postgrad Med J* 1985;61:545–547.

98. Gerding DN, Larson TA, Hughes RA, et al. Aminoglycoside resistance and aminoglycoside usage: ten years of experience in one hospital. *Antimicrob Agents Chemother* 1991;35: 1284–1290.

99. Mollering R Jr. Clinical microbiology and the in vitro activity of aminoglycosides. In: Whelton A, Neu HC, eds. *The aminoglycosides: microbiology, clinical use and toxicology.* New York: Marcel Dekker, 1982:65–95.

100. Sirot D. Extended-spectrum plasmid-mediated beta-lactamases. *J Antimicrob Chemother* 1995;36[Suppl. A]: 19–34.

NEUROLOGY

1. Once diabetes mellitus (DM) and multiple nerve compression injuries have been excluded, the presence of **mononeuritis multiplex** suggests vasculitis. The next question becomes which type. Polyarteritis nodosa is the most common of the vasculitides associated with mononeuritis multiplex, followed by Wegener granulomatosis and Churg-Strauss syndrome (1).

2. Neurologic findings in **vitamin B$_{12}$ deficiency** range from numbness and paresthesias in the extremities (earliest finding), to lower extremity weakness, sensory ataxia, and sphincter abnormalities. Other findings include diminished or increased reflexes, diminished position and vibratory function, subtle personality change, dementia, and psychosis. The neurologic sequelae of B$_{12}$ deficiency can rarely occur with normal hematocrit (2).

3. **Chronic, recurrent meningitis** describes episodes of meningitis with resolution of symptoms, signs, and cerebrospinal fluid (CSF) abnormalities in between the paroxysms. The likely diagnoses include infection with herpes simplex virus II (less likely type I), chemical meningitis from leak of an epidermoid tumor, craniopharyngioma/cholesteatoma, Behçet syndrome, Vogt-Koyanagi-Harada syndrome, systemic lupus erythematosus (SLE), Mollaret meningitis, and drug hypersensitivity to nonsteroidal antiinflammatory drugs. Note: a separate differential diagnosis is used for chronic persistent meningitis (3).

4. **Guillain-Barré syndrome (GBS)** or acute inflammatory demyelinating polyneuropathy often presents

2–4 weeks after a gastroenteritis or upper respiratory infection prodrome. It is manifested by distal paresthesias, ascending paralysis, autonomic dysfunction in 50% of patients, and, in some cases, respiratory compromise from diaphragmatic weakness. *Campylobacter jejuni* is the organism most commonly implicated, and 70% of patients with GBS and *C. jejuni* cultured from their stool recall diarrhea within 12 weeks of the onset of the neuropathy. The diagnosis is established by electrophysiologic studies showing a demyelinating polyneuropathy. The CSF in patients with GBS reveals an elevated protein with few cells, the so-called "albuminocytologic dissociation." Occasionally, axonal pathology predominates, which usually signals a worse prognosis. A pleocytosis in the CSF should prompt other diagnoses (e.g., SLE, sarcoid, and human immunodeficiency virus). The **Miller-Fisher variant** of GBS is the triad of ataxia, ophthalmoplegia, and polyneuropathy. The current treatments of choice are plasma exchange and intravenous immunoglobulin (IVIG). Steroids have no role (4,5).

5. **Creutzfeldt-Jakob disease** should be suspected in persons presenting with rapidly progressive dementia and myoclonus. It can now be diagnosed on the basis of the 14-3-3 protein in the CSF (6).

6. The combination of paroxysmal, severe abdominal pain, motor neuropathy, and neuropsychiatric features suggests the diagnosis of **acute intermittent porphyria (AIP)**. This disease is common in Great Britain and Scandinavia and should be considered when porphyrinogenic stimulants (e.g., alcohol, antiepileptic medications) or gonadal steroids trigger episodes of unexplained abdominal pain. The neuropathy is primarily motor related and often initially causes proximal, upper extremity muscle weakness. Neuropsychiatric manifestations range from depression or paranoia to seizures that can be difficult to control because many antiseizure medications worsen AIP (7,8).

7. Do not forget to examine the eyes of adults who present with a unilateral "worst headache of their life" as-

sociated with nausea and vomiting. The eye examination may reveal a unilateral mid-dilated pupil, sluggishly reactive to light, with a large cup-to-disc ratio and slightly cloudy cornea. An emergent referral to ophthalmology should be made for treatment of **acute angle-closure glaucoma** (9).

8. **Transverse myelitis** should be considered in a patient who presents with rapidly evolving paraparesis, sensory level on the trunk, bowel or bladder incontinence, and up-going toes. CSF findings may be normal early in the course but typically reveal modestly elevated protein with a pleocytosis. Most cases are associated with multiple sclerosis (MS), although postinfectious, postvaccination (particularly hepatitis B), connective tissue diseases (particularly SLE) and paraneoplastic conditions need to be ruled out (10,11).

9. **Bilateral Bell palsy** in a patient from an area endemic with the deer tick *Ixodes dammini* (scapularis) is Lyme disease until proved otherwise. However, other diagnoses that should be entertained include GBS and a form of sarcoidosis known as "Heerfordt syndrome" (uveoparotid fever) (12).

10. The three most likely otologic causes of **peripheral vertigo** are benign paroxysmal positional vertigo (BPPV), vestibular neuronitis (labyrinthitis), and Ménière disease (characterized by episodes of recurrent tinnitus, hearing loss, and vertigo).

11. It is important to distinguish **light-headedness** secondary to orthostatic hypotension from BPPV. Both can cause the patient to feel "dizzy" when standing. Ask the patient to perform movements that will not affect the blood pressure (e.g., head turning or rolling to one side while supine). If the dizziness is reproducible, BPPV is the more likely diagnosis. Orthostasis usually does not cause vertigo (13).

12. Third cranial nerve infarct secondary to DM and microvascular disease typically causes impaired movement of the ipsilateral eye and **spares pupillary function**, whereas aneurysmal compression on the third cranial nerve results in pupillary dilation (14–17).

13. The most common type of diabetic polyradiculopathy is **diabetic amyotrophy**, which classically involves the lumbar roots (L2, L3, and L4). Clinical features include severe, unilateral thigh pain followed by asymmetric thigh weakness in a diabetic. Electromyogram (EMG) can confirm the presence of denervation. The opposite extremity can be affected in some cases (18).

14. The acute onset of **cerebellar ataxia** in an otherwise healthy young adult (no ethanol ingestion) should raise the possibility of MS. Features of nystagmus, scanning speech, and intention tremor known as "Charcot triad," add further to support this diagnosis (19,20).

15. **Vogt-Koyanagi-Harada** syndrome is diagnosed by the clinical manifestations of recurrent aseptic meningitis, uveitis, cranial nerve VIII damage, alopecia, vitiligo, and poliosis (white patch of hair). This disease is more common in Asia (i.e., Japan) than in the United States (21).

16. Patients who present with the insidious onset of myelopathy (bilateral lower extremity weakness, hyperactive deep tendon reflexes, back pain, and urinary incontinence), who have traveled to southwestern Japan or the Caribbean basin (particularly if they have had sexual contact, blood transfusions or injection drug use), should be suspected of having **human T-cell leukemia virus (HTLV-1)-associated myelopathy** (22).

17. **Inclusion body myositis (IBM)** should be considered in patients who present with symmetric muscle weakness and an inflammatory myopathy on EMG testing. IBM is classically seen in patients greater than 50 years of age, may have an insidious onset, and may affect both proximal and distal muscle groups. It can look similar to polymyositis and may be distinguishable only on muscle biopsy that demonstrates rimmed vacuoles and inclusion bodies. A patient diagnosed with polymyositis who does not improve with corticosteroids should raise the possibility of IBM (23).

18. **Myasthenia gravis (MG)** should be suspected when women in their third and fourth decade or men greater than 60 years of age present with easy fatigability, especially in relation to specific muscle groups (e.g., difficulty combing hair or difficulty climbing stairs). Ocular involvement with ptosis, diplopia, or extraocular muscle weakness makes the diagnosis of MG more likely. Other diseases can mimic MG. **Amyotrophic lateral sclerosis** has fasciculations and hyperreflexia that are absent in MG. **Lambert-Eaton syndrome** presents with similar muscle weakness but improves with exercise, a feature not seen in MG. **Botulism** has a more rapid onset and affects the pupils, whereas MG spares the pupils. **Graves disease** can manifest as ophthalmoplegia and weakness, but classically has proptosis and hyperadrenergic features distinct from MG (24–27).

19. The findings of ophthalmoplegia, nystagmus, disorientation, or gait abnormalities (often a slow, wide-based gait) in an alcoholic should point to the possibility of Wernicke encephalopathy. The mainstay of treatment is thiamine. As these symptoms improve, the patient may have difficulty with recent memory and confabulation, which suggests Korsakoff psychosis, a less-reversible feature of the **Wernicke-Korsakoff syndrome**. The pupils are usually spared in this entity, and polyneuropathy likely secondary to nutritional deficiency is present in most cases (28–31).

20. **Normal pressure hydrocephalus (NPH)** is a dementia syndrome that presents with the triad of gait apraxia (magnetic gait where patient has difficulty lifting the feet off the floor), urinary incontinence, and dementia. This triad is not specific for NPH because elderly patients with Alzheimer disease manifest many of these features. The Miller-Fisher test may assist with the diagnosis. Ask the patient to walk a set distance and time the response, then perform a lumbar puncture and withdraw 30 ml of spinal fluid. If the walking pace increases, this strengthens the diagnosis of NPH and

may assist in identifying a subset of patients who will respond to a ventriculoperitoneal shunt (31).

21. An **acoustic neuroma** is a tumor that arises from the vestibular division of the eighth cranial nerve. The acoustic division, however, is damaged more easily than the vestibular division and, therefore, this tumor presents with unilateral hearing loss and, typically, not debilitating dizziness or vertigo. Unilateral hearing loss of unknown cause always deserves evaluation for the presence of this tumor (32).

22. If a patient presents with a **red eye**, one way to differentiate acute conjunctivitis from acute iritis by history is to ask if photophobia is present. Patients with conjunctivitis may complain of a gritty sensation in the eye but they sit in the waiting room with both eyes open. This is in contrast to those with acute iritis, who often cover the affected eye secondary to light sensitivity (33,34).

23. **Parkinson disease** is an illness characterized by tremor, bradykinesia, rigidity, and gait disturbances. The tremor of Parkinson usually begins unilaterally; bilateral tremor on initial presentation weighs heavily against idiopathic Parkinson disease. Patients with idiopathic Parkinson disease usually have at least temporary improvement in symptoms with a trial of L-dopa. No response to this treatment should bring the original diagnosis in to question (35). Progressive supranuclear palsy and drug-induced Parkinsonism are the most commonly confused diagnoses (36).

24. **Internuclear ophthalmoplegia (INO)** represents a delay or loss of movement of the adducting eye on horizontal gaze, with concomitant nystagmus of the abducting eye. With bilateral INO, MS is the most likely diagnosis, although it can manifest (rarely) in Wernicke encephalopathy (37).

25. Weakness secondary to **MG** can be difficult to differentiate from weakness from the side effect of **anticholinesterases** used to treat MG. Drug-induced weakness is usually associated with excessive cholin-

ergic symptoms (e.g., salivation, lacrimation, urination, and defecation). If increasing the anticholinesterase dose in a patient suspected of having a myasthenia crisis, leads to progressive weakness, discontinuation of the medication may be a solution (38,39).

26. A patient who develops weakness and ptosis on penicillamine should be suspected of having **drug-induced myasthenia**. This adverse drug reaction occurs in approximately 1% of patients (40).

REFERENCES

1. Hellmann DB, Laing TJ, Petri M, et al. Mononeuritis multiplex: the yield of evaluations for occult rheumatic diseases. *Medicine (Baltimore)* 1988;67:145–153.
2. Toh BH, van Driel IR, Gleeson PA. Pernicious anemia [see comments]. *N Engl J Med* 1997;337:1441–1448.
3. Coyle PK. Overview of acute and chronic meningitis. *Neurol Clin* 1999;17:691–710.
4. Case records of the Massachusetts General Hospital. Case 39-1999. A 74-year-old woman with acute, progressive paralysis after diarrhea for one week [clinical conference]. *N Engl J Med* 1999;341:1996–2003.
5. Ropper AH. The Guillain-Barré syndrome. *N Engl J Med* 1992; 326:1130–1136.
6. Case records of the Massachusetts General Hospital. Weekly clinicopathological exercises. Case 28-1999. A 68-year-old woman with rapidly progressive dementia and a gait disorder [clinical conference]. *N Engl J Med* 1999;341:901–908.
7. Chen CC, Thajeb P, Lie SK. Acute intermittent porphyria: clinical analysis of nine cases. *Chung Hua I Hsueh Tsa Chih (Taipei)* 1994;54:395–399.
8. Suarez JI, Cohen ML, Larkin J, et al. Acute intermittent porphyria: clinicopathologic correlation. Report of a case and review of the literature [see comments]. *Neurology* 1997;48: 1678–1683.
9. Newman LC, Lipton RB. Emergency department evaluation of headache. *Neurol Clin* 1998;16:285–303.
10. Jeffery DR, Mandler RN, Davis LE. Transverse myelitis. Retrospective analysis of 33 cases, with differentiation of cases associated with multiple sclerosis and parainfectious events. *Arch Neurol* 1993;50:532–535.
11. Thomas M, Thomas J, Jr. Acute transverse myelitis. *J La State Med Soc* 1997;149:75–77.

12. Christen HJ, Bartlau N, Hanefeld F, et al. Peripheral facial palsy in childhood—Lyme borreliosis to be suspected unless proven otherwise. *Acta Paediatr Scand* 1990;79:1219–1224.

13. Furman JM, Cass SP. Benign paroxysmal positional vertigo. *N Engl J Med* 1999;341:1590–1596.

14. Teuscher AU, Meienberg O. Ischaemic oculomotor nerve palsy. Clinical features and vascular risk factors in 23 patients. *J Neurol* 1985;232:144–149.

15. Jacobson DM, McCanna TD, Layde PM. Risk factors for ischemic ocular motor nerve palsies. *Arch Ophthalmol* 1994; 112:961–966.

16. Trobe JD. Isolated pupil-sparing third nerve palsy. *Ophthalmology* 1985;92:58–61.

17. Byrnes DP. Head injury and the dilated pupil. *Am Surg* 1979;45:139–143.

18. Sander HW, Chokroverty S. Diabetic amyotrophy: current concepts. *Semin Neurol* 1996;16:173–178.

19. Ostermann PO, Westerberg CE. Paroxysmal attacks in multiple sclerosis. *Brain* 1975;98:189–202.

20. Rolak LA. The diagnosis of multiple sclerosis. *Neurol Clin* 1996;14:27–43.

21. Perry HD, Font RL. Clinical and histopathologic observations in severe Vogt-Koyanagi-Harada syndrome. *Am J Ophthalmol* 1977;83:242–254.

22. Brew BJ, Price RW. Another retroviral disease of the nervous system: chronic progressive myelopathy due to HTLV-1 [Editorial]. *N Engl J Med* 1988;318:1195–1197.

23. Dalakas MC. Polymyositis, dermatomyositis and inclusion-body myositis [see comments]. *N Engl J Med* 1991;325: 1487–1498.

24. Case records of the Massachusetts General Hospital. Weekly clinicopathological exercises. Case 15-2000. A 69-year-old man with myasthenia gravis and a mediastinal mass [clinical conference]. *N Engl J Med* 2000;342:1508–1514.

25. Drachman DB. Myasthenia gravis. *N Engl J Med* 1994;330: 1797–1810.

26. Williams DB, Windebank AJ. Motor neuron disease (amyotrophic lateral sclerosis). *Mayo Clin Proc* 1991;66:54–82.

27. Case records of the Massachusetts General Hospital. Weekly clinicopathological exercises. Case 32-1994. A 61-year-old man with muscular weakness [clinical conference] [published erratum appears in *N Engl J Med* 1994;331(24):1667]. *N Engl J Med* 1994;331:528–535.

28. Wood B, Currie J, Breen K. Wernicke's encephalopathy in a metropolitan hospital. A prospective study of incidence, characteristics and outcome [published erratum appears in *Med J Aust* 1986;144(5):280]. *Med J Aust* 1986;144:12–16.

29. Reuler JB, Girard DE, Cooney TG. Current concepts. Wernicke's encephalopathy. *N Engl J Med* 1985;312:1035–1039.
30. Zubaran C, Fernandes JG, Rodnight R. Wernicke-Korsakoff syndrome. *Postgrad Med J* 1997;73:27–31.
31. Vanneste JA. Diagnosis and management of normal-pressure hydrocephalus. *J Neurol* 2000;247:5–14.
32. Spoelhof GD. When to suspect an acoustic neuroma. *Am Fam Physician* 1995;52:1768–1774.
33. Morrow GL, Abbott RL. Conjunctivitis [see comments]. *Am Fam Physician* 1998;57:735–746.
34. Hara JH. The red eye: diagnosis and treatment. *Am Fam Physician* 1996;54:2423–2430.
35. Lang AE, Lozano AM. Parkinson's disease. Second of two parts. *N Engl J Med* 1998;339:1130–1143.
36. Lang AE, Lozano AM. Parkinson's disease. First of two parts. *N Engl J Med* 1998;339:1044–1053.
37. De La Paz MA, Chung SM, McCrary JA, III. Bilateral internuclear ophthalmoplegia in a patient with Wernicke's encephalopathy. *J Clin Neuroophthalmol* 1992;12:116–120.
38. Heitmiller RF.Myasthenia gravis: clinical features, pathogenesis, evaluation, and medical management. *Semin Thorac Cardiovasc Surg* 1999;11:41–46.
39. O'Riordan JI, Miller DH, Mottershead JP, et al. The management and outcome of patients with myasthenia gravis treated acutely in a neurological intensive care unit. *Eur J Neurol* 1998;5:137–142.
40. Raynauld JP, Lee YS, Kornfeld P, et al. Unilateral ptosis as an initial manifestation of D-penicillamine induced myasthenia gravis. *J Rheumatol* 1993;20:1592–1593.

9

ONCOLOGY

1. Certain patients who fulfill the criteria for **cancer of unknown primary site (CUPS)** tend to be more responsive to cisplatin-based chemotherapy. Features include poorly differentiated carcinoma; age less than 50 years; tumor involving midline structures, lung parenchyma, or lymph nodes; elevated serum α-fetoprotein (AFP) or β-human chorionic gonadotropin; rapid tumor growth; cancer previously responsive to chemotherapy or radiation, or favorable performance status around the time of initial diagnosis. Many of these features are consistent with poorly differentiated germ cell tumor. Of the patients who present with CUPS and poorly differentiated carcinoma who are treated with chemotherapy aimed against germ cell tumors, one fourth will respond completely and one third will have a partial response (1).

2. The most common neoplasm responsible for **superior vena cava (SVC) syndrome** is small cell lung cancer followed by lymphoma (Hodgkin disease and non-Hodgkin's lymphoma) (2–4).

3. A **Virchow sentinel node** (left supraclavicular lymph node) raises the possibility of gastric cancer. Other gastrointestinal (GI) malignancies associated with Virchow node include colon cancer, pancreatic cancer, renal cell carcinoma, testicular, ovarian, and prostate cancer. A right supraclavicular node should suggest the possibility of lung cancer, esophageal cancer, or cancer involving the mediastinum (5).

4. **Tumor lysis syndrome** should be considered in a patient with underlying neoplasm who develops renal

failure with high levels of uric acid and hyperphosphatemia. It is associated in particular with treatment of high-grade lymphomas, Burkitt lymphoma, and acute lymphoblastic leukemia. In addition, a spontaneous form may develop in the absence of chemotherapy. The two forms can be differentiated because spontaneous tumor lysis syndrome may not present with hyperphosphatemia (6).

5. The most common malignancy associated with dermatomyositis in women is **ovarian cancer** (7).

6. Suspect **multiple myeloma** in any middle-aged or elderly patient with bone pain, unexplained anemia, unexplained renal insufficiency (bland urine sediment without proteinuria), hypercalcemia, increased frequency of infections with encapsulated bacteria, lytic bone lesions found on skeletal survey, hypoalbuminemia with increased total protein, positive serum protein electrophoresis, and increased Bence Jones proteins in the urine. A plasmacytoma or bone marrow biopsy with greater than 10% plasma cells makes the diagnosis of multiple myeloma more likely (8).

7. The finding of black cerebrospinal fluid is pathognomonic for **primary spinal melanoma** (9,10)

8. A syndrome of "dancing eyes-dancing feet," termed **opsoclonus-myoclonus** is seen in children with neuroblastomas. In adults, this syndrome may be associated with solid tumors (e.g., bronchial cancer). Some women present with breast cancer and paraneoplastic opsoclonus in association with anti-Ri antibodies (RNA-binding proteins) (11).

9. **Peritoneal carcinomatosis** in a woman with pathologic findings demonstrating adenocarcinoma of unknown primary site should be treated as ovarian cancer (12–14).

10. A history of head or neck irradiation, vocal cord paralysis, or enlarged regional lymph nodes in the setting of a **thyroid nodule** increases the likelihood of malignancy (15,16).

11. **Anti-Hu antibodies** have been documented in patients who present with paraneoplastic sensory neuropathy, encephalomyelitis, and opsoclonus–myoclonus. Anti-Hu refers to neuron-specific RNA binding nuclear proteins, which are most often seen in the setting of small cell carcinoma of the lung (17,18).

12. Patients with underlying **asbestosis** have an increased risk of lung cancer. The risk of lung cancer increases even further with tobacco use (19,20).

13. **Pancoast syndrome** is most commonly caused by superior sulcus tumors, especially non—small-cell lung tumors. The most common clinical manifestations of this syndrome are shoulder pain, arm pain (distribution of dermatome C8, T1, and T2), hand atrophy, and Horner syndrome which is the triad of miosis, ptosis, and anhidrosis (21).

14. Oncology patients who present with signs and symptoms of congestive heart failure and describe a history of chemotherapy use increases the likelihood of **anthracycline-induced cardiomyopathy**. Most of these cases occur in patients who have received greater than 500 mg/m^2 of anthracycline (22).

15. **Fibrolamellar variant of hepatocellular carcinoma (HCC)** is much less common but has a better prognosis than HCC. It is not associated with underlying cirrhosis. AFP is not helpful in the diagnosis because the tumor does not secrete AFP (23).

16. **Acral lentiginous melanoma** is a type of cutaneous melanoma that is more common in blacks and affects non—sun-exposed areas of skin, including palms and soles (24,25).

17. Conditions that predispose to **angiosarcoma** are drugs (thorotrast, polyvinyl chloride), external beam therapeutic radiation, and chronic lymphedema (26–28).

18. **Pancreatic cancer** often presents with abdominal or back pain, weight loss, anorexia, painless jaundice, pruritus, and migratory superficial thrombophlebitis. For reasons not entirely clear, some of these patients will have symptoms of depression before their

diagnosis, which may serve as a clue to the site of their cancer (29,30).

19. Patients who present with multiple cutaneous hamartomas may have **Cowden syndrome**. There is a high incidence of thyroid cancer and, in particular, breast cancer. The association with breast cancer is so strong that prophylactic mastectomy is often necessary (31,32)

20. The three most common primary malignancies that **metastasize** to the **adrenal glands** are lung cancer, breast cancer, and melanoma (33–35).

21. Two primary brain tumors **cross the corpus callosum**: glioblastoma multiforme and primary central nervous system lymphoma (36,37).

22. Solid tumors that have a predilection to **metastasize to bone** are carcinomas of the prostate, lung, breast, kidney, and thyroid (38–41).

23. **Prostate cancer** rarely metastasizes to the brain. In a patient who is known to have underlying prostate cancer and newly discovered brain masses, consider the possibility of a second primary cancer (42).

24. Facial swelling and a history of malignancy suggest **superior vena cava (SVC) syndrome** (43).

25. The liver inactivates the secretory products of carcinoid tumors, which may explain why carcinoid tumors of the GI tract will cause the **carcinoid syndrome** only if hepatic metastases are present (44).

REFERENCES

1. Lembersky BC, Thomas LC. Metastases of unknown primary site. *Med Clin North Am* 1996;80:153–171.
2. Kovacs RG, Aguayo SM. Images in clinical medicine. Superior vena cava syndrome [see comments]. *N Engl J Med* 1993;329:1007.
3. Nieto AF, Doty DB. Superior vena cava obstruction: clinical syndrome, etiology, and treatment. *Curr Probl Cancer* 1986; 10:441–484.
4. Mineo TC, Ambrogi V, Nofroni I, et al. Mediastinoscopy in superior vena cava obstruction: analysis of 80 consecutive patients. *Ann Thorac Surg* 1999;68:223–226.

5. McHenry CR, Cooney MM, Slusarczyk SJ, et al. Supraclavicular lymphadenopathy: the spectrum of pathology and evaluation by fine-needle aspiration biopsy. *Am Surg* 1999;65: 742–746.
6. Jasek AM, Day HJ. Acute spontaneous tumor lysis syndrome. *Am J Hematol* 1994;47:129–131.
7. Callen JP. Dermatomyositis [see comments]. *Lancet* 2000; 355:53–57.
8. Bataille R, Harousseau JL. Multiple myeloma. *N Engl J Med* 1997;336:1657–1664.
9. Gokaslan ZL, Aladag MA, Ellerhorst JA. Melanoma metastatic to the spine: a review of 133 cases. *Melanoma Res* 2000; 10:78–80.
10. Spiegel DA, Sampson JH, Richardson WJ, et al. Metastatic melanoma to the spine. Demographics, risk factors, and prognosis in 114 patients. *Spine* 1995;20:2141–2146.
11. Connolly AM, Pestronk A, Mehta S, et al. Serum autoantibodies in childhood opsoclonus-myoclonus syndrome: an analysis of antigenic targets in neural tissues [see comments]. *J Pediatr* 1997;130:878–884.
12. Della-Fiorentina SA, Jaworski RC, Crandon AJ, et al. Primary peritoneal carcinoma: a treatable subset of patients with adenocarcinoma of unknown primary. *Aust N Z J Surg* 1996;66: 124–125.
13. Sporn JR, Greenberg BR. Empirical chemotherapy for adenocarcinoma of unknown primary tumor site. *Semin Oncol* 1993;20:261–267.
14. Strnad CM, Grosh WW, Baxter J, et al. Peritoneal carcinomatosis of unknown primary site in women. A distinctive subset of adenocarcinoma. *Ann Intern Med* 1989;111:213–217.
15. Belfiore A, La Rosa GL, La Porta GA, et al. Cancer risk in patients with cold thyroid nodules: relevance of iodine intake, sex, age, and multinodularity [see comments]. *Am J Med* 1992;93:363–369.
16. Schlumberger MJ. Papillary and follicular thyroid carcinoma. *N Engl J Med* 1998;338:297–306.
17. King PH, Redden D, Palmgren JS, et al. Hu antigen specificities of ANNA-I autoantibodies in paraneoplastic neurological disease. *J Autoimmun* 1999;13:435–443.
18. Verschuuren JJ, Perquin M, ten Velde G, et al. Anti-Hu antibody titre and brain metastases before and after treatment for small cell lung cancer. *J Neurol Neurosurg Psychiatry* 1999; 67:353–357.
19. Billings CG, Howard P. Asbestos exposure, lung cancer and asbestosis. *Monaldi Arch Chest Dis* 2000;55:151–156.
20. Boffetta P. Health effects of asbestos exposure in humans: a quantitative assessment. *Med Lav* 1998;89:471–480.

21. Hilaris BS, Martini N, Wong GY, et al. Treatment of superior sulcus tumor (Pancoast tumor). *Surg Clin North Am* 1987;67: 965–977.

22. Fisher NG, Marshall AJ. Anthracycline-induced cardiomyopathy. *Postgrad Med J* 1999;75:265–268.

23. Wetzel WJ, Costin JL, Petrino RL. Fibrolamellar carcinoma: distinctive clinical and morphologic variant of hepatoma. *South Med J* 1983;76:796–798.

24. Zimmerman GC, Grabski WJ. Images in clinical medicine. Malignant melanoma. *N Engl J Med* 1994;331:168.

25. Hudson DA, Krige JE, Stubbings H. Plantar melanoma: results of treatment in three population groups. *Surgery* 1998; 124:877–882.

26. Doll R. Effects of exposure to vinyl chloride. An assessment of the evidence. *Scand J Work Environ Health* 1988;14:61–78.

27. Kielhorn J, Melber C, Wahnschaffe U, et al. Vinyl chloride: still a cause for concern. *Environ Health Perspect* 2000;108: 579–588.

28. Majeski J, Austin RM, Fitzgerald RH. Cutaneous angiosarcoma in an irradiated breast after breast conservation therapy for cancer: association with chronic breast lymphedema. *J Surg Oncol* 2000;74:208–212.

29. Warshaw AL, Fernandez-del Castillo C. Pancreatic carcinoma. *N Engl J Med* 1992;326:455–465.

30. Joffe RT, Rubinow DR, Denicoff KD, et al. Depression and carcinoma of the pancreas. *Gen Hosp Psychiatry* 1986;8: 241–245.

31. Case records of the Massachusetts General Hospital. Weekly clinicopathological exercises. Case 24-1987. A 56-year-old man with a substernal goiter, multiple cutaneous and mucosal lesions, and a positive stool test for occult blood. *N Engl J Med* 1987;316:1531–1540.

32. Katz SK, Gordon KB, Roenigk HH. The cutaneous manifestations of gastrointestinal disease. *Prim Care* 1996;23:455–476.

33. Miyaji N, Miki T, Itoh Y, et al. Radiotherapy for adrenal gland metastasis from lung cancer: report of three cases. *Radiat Med* 1999;17:71–75.

34. Haigh PI, Essner R, Wardlaw JC, et al. Long-term survival after complete resection of melanoma metastatic to the adrenal gland [see comments]. *Ann Surg Oncol* 1999;6: 633–639.

35. Aldrete JS, Bohrod MG. Adrenal metastases in cancer of the breast. Their prognostic significance when found at adrenalectomy. *Am Surg* 1967;33:174–178.

36. Blumenthal DT, DeAngelis LM. Aging and primary central nervous system neoplasms. *Neurol Clin* 1998;16:671–686.

37. Forsyth PA, DeAngelis LM. Biology and management of AIDS-associated primary CNS lymphomas. *Hematol Oncol Clin North Am* 1996;10:1125–1134.
38. Plunkett TA, Rubens RD. The biology and management of bone metastases. *Crit Rev Oncol Hematol* 1999;31:89–96.
39. Onimus M, Papin P, Gangloff S. Results of surgical treatment of spinal thoracic and lumbar metastases. *Eur Spine J* 1996; 5:407–411.
40. Goldman FD, Dayton PD, Hanson CJ. Renal cell carcinoma and osseous metastases. Case report and literature review. *J Am Podiatr Med Assoc* 1989;79:618–625.
41. Pittas AG, Adler M, Fazzari M, et al. Bone metastases from thyroid carcinoma: clinical characteristics and prognostic variables in one hundred forty-six patients. *Thyroid* 2000;10: 261–268.
42. Fervenza FC, Wolanskyj AP, Eklund HE, et al. Brain metastasis: an unusual complication from prostatic adenocarcinoma. *Mayo Clin Proc* 2000;75:79–82.
43. Kelly KM, Lange B. Oncologic emergencies. *Pediatr Clin North Am* 1997;44:809–830.
44. Kulke MH, Mayer RJ. Carcinoid tumors [see comments]. *N Engl J Med* 1999;340:858–868.

10

PULMONARY

1. Congestive heart failure (CHF), pulmonary infections, malignancy, and pulmonary thromboembolism account for 90% of all **pleural effusions**. When the effusion is exudative, pulmonary infections and malignancy are the most common causes (1–3).

2. **Allergic bronchopulmonary aspergillosis (ABPA)** should be considered in a patient with underlying asthma refractory to treatment, asthma complicated by fleeting pulmonary infiltrates seen on a chest x-ray study, eosinophilia beyond what is normally expected for asthma (5% to 10%), expectoration of brownish mucous plugs, hemoptysis, or central bronchiectasis on high-resolution computed tomography (HRCT) scan. Asthma and ABPA are highly associated and the absence of underlying asthma makes ABPA less likely (4).

3. When persistent fevers are caused by **sarcoidosis**, sarcoid has usually infiltrated the liver. The most common laboratory abnormality is an elevated alkaline phosphatase (5).

4. In patients considered to have **bilateral diaphragmatic muscle weakness** from either motor neuron disease, neuropathies, or myopathies, a useful test to assist in diagnosis is supine and upright vital capacity (VC) pulmonary function tests. In the normal patient, VC should remain the same or decrease by less than 10% when converting from the upright to supine position. In patients with diaphragmatic paralysis, VC may decrease in the supine position 50% or more (6,7).

5. Several clinical and historical clues exist to diagnose
    asbestosis. It is important to document asbestos ex-
    posure, which should have been in the distant past to
    allow for the proper clinical latency of the disease.
    Common symptoms include breathlessness and non-
    productive cough. On examination, bilateral crackles
    may be auscultated. Interstitial radiographic changes
    can be seen on chest x-ray study or HRCT. The radio-
    graphic hallmark of asbestosis is pleural disease.
    Pleural plaques are almost pathognomonic of prior ex-
    posure. Interstitial reticulonodular infiltrates usually
    begin at the bases. This is one of the few chronic
    interstitial lung diseases with pleural involvement.
    Restrictive lung disease is the rule and pulmonary
    function tests demonstrate decreased diffusing capac-
    ity of lung for carbon monoxide (D_{LCO}) and decreased
    total lung capacity. Asbestos bodies can be visualized
    by bronchoscopy with bronchoalveolar lavage (BAL)
    or biopsy, but this is often unnecessary (8).

6. The acute onset of shortness of breath and bilateral
    patchy pulmonary infiltrates in a patient who has re-
    cently received a transfusion of blood products should
    raise the suspicion of **transfusion-related acute lung
    injury**. The differential diagnosis includes intravascu-
    lar volume overload (cardiomegaly may be a clue) and
    acute hemolytic reaction (9).

7. Although occurring in less than 50% of patients, head,
    neck, chest, or axillary petechiae in a hypoxemic
    patient with prior long bone fractures should strongly
    suggest the diagnosis of **fat embolism syndrome**
    (10–12).

8. Cystic fibrosis (CF) and ABPA are two diseases that
    cause **bronchiectasis**. HRCT scanning may help
    differentiate the two. CF tends to cause diffuse upper
    lobe bronchiectasis, whereas central bronchiectasis
    is more specific for ABPA. It is important to remem-
    ber that some patients can have both diseases (13).

9. S1Q3T3 is an uncommon electrocardiographic (ECG)
    finding of **acute pulmonary embolism (PE)**. Two

more common ECG abnormalities in acute PE are sinus tachycardia and T-wave inversions in the anteroseptal precordial leads (14).

10. The most common clinical manifestations of **pleural mesothelioma** are shortness of breath and nonpleuritic chest pain. Men are affected more commonly than women and are usually in their fifth to seventh decade of life. The most common radiographic presentation is a large, unilateral pleural effusion. Diagnosis can rarely be made by thoracentesis, although thoracoscopic pleural biopsy greatly enhances the diagnostic yield (15–17).

11. **Pulmonary silicosis** increases the risk of pulmonary and extrapulmonary tuberculosis, as well as the mortality from TB (18).

12. Chronic respiratory symptoms and a chest x-ray study that shows bilateral peripheral infiltrates, the photo-negative of CHF, should raise suspicion for **eosinophilic pneumonia** (19).

13. **Pulmonary eosinophilic granuloma**, a subtype of histiocytosis X, is one of few disease processes that can present with simultaneous, bilateral spontaneous pneumothoraces (20).

14. The triad of shortness of breath, pleuritic chest pain, and hemoptysis should lead to the consideration of **pulmonary embolism (PE)** with **infarction**. Those who present with this triad and neutropenia should be investigated for **invasive aspergillosis** (21,22).

15. **Acute eosinophilic pneumonia** typically presents with fever, nonproductive cough, bilateral interstitial infiltrates, peripheral eosinophilia (occasionally), eosinophilia on BAL, and no other obvious cause of pneumonia. This disease is exquisitely sensitive to glucocorticoids, and the absence of clinical improvement within a day or two should suggest an alternative diagnosis (23).

16. The right ventricular systolic pressure (RVSP) usually does not exceed 40 mm Hg in cases of an **acute**

PE in a patient with a previously normal cardio-vascular system. The finding of an RVSP greater than 40 mm Hg by echocardiography implies either chronic pulmonary hypertension or an acute on chronic process (24).

17. Any process that disrupts the integrity of the thoracic duct can cause a **chylothorax**. The two most common causes of which are surgery and malignancies. Lymphoma is the most common underlying malignancy. Chylothorax should be suspected in any patient with milky color pleural fluid rich in chylomicrons, although chylothoraces can be seen with serosanguinous or bloody effusions. A pleural fluid triglyceride greater than 110 mg/dl strongly supports this diagnosis, whereas a level less than 50 mg/dl rules out the possibility of chylothorax (25,26).

18. **Aspiration pneumonia** classically targets the superior segment of lower lobes in patients who aspirate while supine (27,28).

19. Patients with underlying **pulmonary alveolar proteinosis (PAP)** have a significantly increased risk of nocardial infection. This gram-positive, weakly acid fast actinomycete should be considered in patients with underlying PAP who decompensate clinically (29).

20. **Alpha-1 antitrypsin deficiency** should be suspected in adults who present with dyspnea in their fourth and fifth decades and radiographic abnormalities that include emphysematous changes predominantly affecting the basilar segments of the lungs. This is in contrast to classic emphysema where the apices typically show emphysematous changes. One point regarding alpha-1 antitrypsin deficiency is smoking can accelerate the onset of the disease by up to 20 years. The liver is the other organ system that may be involved (30).

21. ***Pseudomonas* (Burkholderia) *cepacia* pneumonia** portends an unfavorable prognosis in patients with underlying CF. It is a contraindication to lung transplantation in *some* centers (31).

22. Clubbing and bilateral lower lobe interstitial pulmonary infiltrates in an adult over 50 years of age is likely to represent **idiopathic pulmonary fibrosis**. Other less likely possibilities include asbestosis, lymphangitic spread of carcinoma, and collagen-vascular disease (32).

23. A patient who presents with insidious, progressive dyspnea on exertion and nonproductive cough with a history significant for lung irradiation may have **radiation pneumonitis**. One clue to this diagnosis radiographically is the straight-line effect that conforms to the boundaries of the prior radiation field (33).

24. Most patients with underlying **sleep apnea** do not suffer from **obesity-hypoventilation syndrome (OHS)**. The opposite is not true. Most patients with OHS have concomitant sleep apnea. Patients with sleep apnea alone do not have significantly elevated Pco_2 on arterial blood gas, as opposed to patients with OHS who, by definition, have elevated arterial Pco_2. The diagnosis of sleep apnea is made by history and sleep study. Obesity, CO_2 retention, and exclusion of other disease processes that cause hypoventilation lead to the diagnosis of OHS (34).

25. A **persistent, unexplained pleural effusion** for greater than 1 year is unusual and limits the differential diagnosis to yellow nail syndrome (yellow nails, lymphedema, and respiratory tract pathology) and trapped lung (i.e., secondary to rheumatoid arthritis or tuberculosis) (35,36).

26. The diagnosis of pulmonary **lymphangioleiomyomatosis** should be considered in any premenopausal woman who presents with shortness of breath and chylothorax. HRCT scan often shows hyperinflated lungs with diffuse, homogenous cystic lesions. These patients are often misdiagnosed as having emphysema (37).

27. In critically ill patients with evidence of a **community-acquired pneumonia** on chest x-ray study, the two organisms that can be rapidly fatal are *Legionella pneumophila* and the pneumococcus (38,39).

28. Dyspnea is the most common feature of **air embolism**, a diagnosis that should be considered in any patient with sudden hemodynamic compromise in the setting of an open communication between the atmosphere and the bloodstream (40).

29. Patients with **diaphragmatic weakness** often relate abrupt onset of dyspnea while in the supine position (41).

30. In the absence of CHF, the most common cause of **bilateral transudative effusions** is ascites (42).

31. Idiopathic **bronchiolitis obliterans with organizing pneumonia** can be challenging to diagnose, but should be considered in patients who present with symptoms of community-acquired pneumonia, nonproductive cough, dyspnea, and weight loss, and do not improve with antibiotics. The most common radiologic abnormality is bilateral alveolar opacities that, at times, have a predilection for the periphery of the lung (similar to eosinophilic pneumonia). Diagnosis can be made definitively only with lung biopsy (43,44).

32. A finding of greater than 10% **mesothelial cells** in pleural fluid makes the diagnosis of pleural tuberculosis highly unlikely (45).

33. Nodules and cystic lesions that predominate in the mid to upper lung zones on chest x-ray study or HRCT, especially in the setting of a tobacco use, is highly suggestive of **pulmonary histiocytosis X (eosinophilic granuloma)**. This disease is often detected in routine screening of asymptomatic adults. The most common symptoms are nonproductive cough and dyspnea. Recurrent pneumothoraces, osteolytic bone lesions, and diabetes insipidus reinforce the diagnosis. Tobacco cessation is the most important therapy (46).

34. Renal artery stenosis should be considered in the differential diagnosis of **flash pulmonary edema** (47,48).

35. Sarcoidosis presenting with polyarthritis, erythema nodosum, and hilar adenopathy is referred to as

Lofgren syndrome, which has an excellent prognosis without systemic corticosteroids. Aspirin often relieves the arthritic pain. This presentation is more common in women with sarcoidosis. The polyarthritis most commonly affects the ankles and knees and can be confused with reactive arthritis. Sarcoidosis should always be listed on the differential diagnosis of seronegative polyarthritis (49).

36. **Hypertrophic pulmonary osteoarthropathy (HPO)**, also known as Bamberger-Pierre Marie syndrome, can be detected clinically by digital clubbing, painful, bilateral periostitis of the tibia and fibula (most commonly), and synovial effusions. The most common neoplasm associated with HPO is bronchogenic carcinoma (most notably adenocarcinoma). HPO can also accompany chronic infections (bronchiectasis, lung abscess, subacute bacterial endocarditis), chronic interstitial pneumonitis, and inflammatory bowel disease. The absence of clubbing makes the diagnosis of HPO less likely (50–52).

37. The differential diagnosis of an **anterior mediastinal mass** includes thymoma, lymphoma, teratoma, mediastinal cysts, and substernal thyroid. Thymoma is the most common cause of an anterior mediastinal mass, followed by lymphoma. A mass in the anterior mediastinum is more likely to be malignant than masses in the middle or posterior compartments (53–55).

38. The triad of lacrimegaly, cough that is responsive only to steroids, and hilar or paratracheal adenopathy suggests **sarcoidosis** (56,57).

39. A patient who becomes dyspneic and desaturates when placed in the upright position should be evaluated for right-to-left shunt. A patent foramen ovale is the most common explanation for a patient who exhibits **platypnea** (dyspnea in the upright position) and **orthodeoxia** (arterial hypoxemia in the upright position), but this phenomenon has also been observed with pneumonectomy, recurrent pulmonary emboli, and pulmonary arteriovenous (AV) malformations (58–60).

40. Occult stroke in a young person should raise suspicion for **pulmonary AV fistula (PAVF)**. More than one third of patients with PAVF have neurologic complications, often in the form of brain abscesses (61,62).

41. It is difficult to discern on chest x-ray study if a peripheral lesion continuous with the chest wall is within the pleura or within the lung parenchyma. An acute angle at the junction between the lesion and the chest wall suggests that the lesion lies within the lung parenchyma, whereas an obtuse angle suggests that the lesion is pleural-based, which is termed the **extrapleural sign** (63).

42. **Samter syndrome** is the triad of bronchial asthma, nasal polyposis, and intolerance to aspirin. Marked eosinophilia is noted in the peripheral blood and respiratory secretions of these patients, and 10% of the patients have urticaria, angioedema, or both. The syndrome is responsive to leukotriene inhibitors, and treatment of the nasal polyps has been shown to improve the patients' asthma (64–67).

43. Classically pleural effusions associated with **PE** are said to be bloody; however, less than 20% of these effusions are bloody. These effusions are highly variable in terms of cellular composition and typically resolve once anticoagulative treatment is started (68).

44. **Pleural fluid eosinophilia** (>10% eosinophils) is most often the result of air or blood within the pleural space. Pneumothorax and trauma are the most common causes, followed by occult pulmonary thromboembolism and benign asbestos effusions. Pleural fluid eosinophilia has no predictive value in terms of malignancy, but does make the diagnosis of tuberculosis unlikely (69,70).

45. The diagnosis of **inhalation fever** (metal fume fever or grain fever) should be considered in industrial workers with rapid onset of intense shaking chills, fever, and body aches while on the job. Inhalation fever is a benign, self-limited process that spontaneously resolves within 24–48 hours after exposure to metallic

fumes ceases. This entity is often misdiagnosed as a viral illness, and can be induced by metal fumes (i.e., zinc oxide), bioaerosols (i.e., grains), and polymer fumes (71,72).

46. A **solitary pulmonary nodule (SPN)** has a low radiographic risk for malignancy on CT scan if the nodule has diffuse or popcorn calcifications, smooth margins with no irregularity, and has been radiographically stable for at least 2 years. In contrast, an SPN greater than 2.5 cm in size with grossly irregular or spiculated margins has a high likelihood of being malignant (73).

47. Drugs that can cause radiographically significant **pulmonary granuloma formation** include talc (illicit heroin use), methotrexate, mineral oil (lipoid granuloma), and bacille Calmette-Guérin vaccine (74).

48. Consider the diagnosis of **berylliosis** in patients suspected of having sarcoidosis, because they have similar respiratory, biochemical, and radiographic features. The clinical history of beryllium exposure (work in the metal or aerospace industry) and the presence of noncaseating pulmonary granuloma help with the diagnosis. A positive blood beryllium lymphocyte proliferation test, however, makes the diagnosis of berylliosis likely (75,76).

49. After a routine thoracentesis, where a pleural biopsy is not taken, the chest x-ray study should be limited to patients with symptoms indicative of **thoracentesis-induced pneumothorax** (77,78).

REFERENCES

1. Prabhudesai PP, Mahashur AA, Mehta N, et al. Exudative pleural effusions in patients over forty years of age–an analysis of seventy-six patients [see comments]. *J Postgrad Med* 1993;39:190–193.
2. Light RW, Macgregor MI, Luchsinger PC, et al. Pleural effusions: the diagnostic separation of transudates and exudates. *Ann Intern Med* 1972;77:507–513.
3. Marel M, Zrustova M, Stasny B, et al. The incidence of pleural effusion in a well-defined region. Epidemiologic study in central Bohemia. *Chest* 1993;104:1486–1489.

4. Cockrill BA, Hales CA. Allergic bronchopulmonary aspergillosis. *Annu Rev Med* 1999;50:303–316.

5. Hercules HD, Bethlem NM. Value of liver biopsy in sarcoidosis. *Arch Pathol Lab Med* 1984;108:831–834.

6. Rochester DF, Esau SA. Assessment of ventilatory function in patients with neuromuscular disease. *Clin Chest Med* 1994;15:751–763.

7. Sandham JD, Shaw DT, Guenter CA. Acute supine respiratory failure due to bilateral diaphragmatic paralysis. *Chest* 1977;72:96–98.

8. Lordi GM, Reichman LB. Pulmonary complications of asbestos exposure [see comments]. *Am Fam Physician* 1993; 48:1471–1477.

9. Kopko PM, Holland PV. Transfusion-related acute lung injury. *Br J Haematol* 1999;105:322–329.

10. Gong H, Jr. Fat embolism syndrome: a puzzling phenomenon. *Postgrad Med* 1977;62:40–48.

11. Gossling HR, Donohue TA. The fat embolism syndrome. *JAMA* 1979;241:2740–2742.

12. Johnson MJ, Lucas GL. Fat embolism syndrome. *Orthopedics* 1996;19:41–48.

13. Cartier Y, Kavanagh PV, Johkoh T, et al. Bronchiectasis: accuracy of high-resolution CT in the differentiation of specific diseases. *AJR* 1999;173:47–52.

14. Ferrari E, Imbert A, Chevalier T, et al. The ECG in pulmonary embolism. Predictive value of negative T waves in precordial leads–80 case reports [see comments]. *Chest* 1997;111: 537–543.

15. Sterman DH, Kaiser LR, Albelda SM. Advances in the treatment of malignant pleural mesothelioma. *Chest* 1999;116: 504–520.

16. Astoul P. Pleural mesothelioma. *Curr Opin Pulm Med* 1999; 5:259–268.

17. Ng CS, Munden RF, Libshitz HI. Malignant pleural mesothelioma: the spectrum of manifestations on CT in 70 cases. *Clin Radiol* 1999;54:415–421.

18. Hnizdo E, Murray J. Risk of pulmonary tuberculosis relative to silicosis and exposure to silica dust in South African gold miners [published erratum appears in *Occup Environ Med* 1999;56(3):215–216]. *Occup Environ Med* 1998;55:496–502.

19. Pope-Harman AL, Davis WB, Allen ED, et al. Acute eosinophilic pneumonia. A summary of 15 cases and review of the literature. *Medicine (Baltimore)* 1996;75:334–342.

20. Graf-Deuel E, Knoblauch A. Simultaneous bilateral spontaneous pneumothorax. *Chest* 1994;105:1142–1146.

21. Bell WR, Simon TL, DeMets DL. The clinical features of submassive and massive pulmonary emboli. *Am J Med* 1977;62: 355–360.

22. Schwartz S, Thiel E. Clinical presentation of invasive aspergillosis. *Mycoses* 1997;40[Suppl. 2]:21–24.

23. Acute eosinophilic pneumonia [see comments]. *Lancet* 1990; 335:947.

24. Come PC. Echocardiographic evaluation of pulmonary embolism and its response to therapeutic interventions. *Chest* 1992;101:151S–162S.

25. Yeam I, Sassoon C. Hemothorax and chylothorax. *Curr Opin Pulm Med* 1997;3:310–314.

26. Miller JI, Jr. Diagnosis and management of chylothorax. *Chest Surg Clin N Am* 1996;6:139–148.

27. Lomotan JR, George SS, Brandstetter RD. Aspiration pneumonia. Strategies for early recognition and prevention. *Postgrad Med* 1997;102:225–231.

28. Finegold SM. Aspiration pneumonia. *Rev Infect Dis* 1991; 13[Suppl. 9]:S737–S742.

29. Pascual J, Gomez Aguinaga MA, Vidal R, et al. Alveolar proteinosis and nocardiosis: a patient treated by bronchopulmonary lavage. *Postgrad Med J* 1989;65:674–677.

30. Perlmutter DH. Alpha-1-antitrypsin deficiency. *Semin Liver Dis* 1998;18:217–225.

31. Hendry J, Elborn JS, Nixon L, et al. Cystic fibrosis: inflammatory response to infection with *Burkholderia cepacia* and *Pseudomonas aeruginosa*. *Eur Respir J* 1999;14:435–438.

32. Kanematsu T, Kitaichi M, Nishimura K, et al. Clubbing of the fingers and smooth-muscle proliferation in fibrotic changes in the lung in patients with idiopathic pulmonary fibrosis. *Chest* 1994;105:339–342.

33. Salinas FV, Winterbauer RH. Radiation pneumonitis: a mimic of infectious pneumonitis. *Semin Respir Infect* 1995;10: 143–153.

34. Rapoport DM, Garay SM, Epstein H, et al. Hypercapnia in the obstructive sleep apnea syndrome. A reevaluation of the "Pickwickian syndrome." *Chest* 1986;89:627–635.

35. Morandi U, Golinelli M, Brandi L, et al. "Yellow nail syndrome" associated with chronic recurrent pericardial and pleural effusions. *Eur J Cardiothorac Surg* 1995;9:42–44.

36. Gea J, Ballester E, Mayordomo C, et al. Trapped lung syndrome. A rare cause of chronic pleural effusion. *Med Clin (Barc)* 1985;84:825–827.

37. Sullivan EJ. Lymphangioleiomyomatosis: a review. *Chest* 1998;114:1689–1703.

38. Moine P, Vercken JB, Chevret S, et al. Severe community-acquired pneumonia. Etiology, epidemiology, and prognosis factors. French Study Group for Community-Acquired Pneumonia in the Intensive Care Unit [see comments]. *Chest* 1994;105:1487–1495.

39. Falco V, Fernandez DS, Alegre J, et al. Legionella pneumophila. A cause of severe community-acquired pneumonia. *Chest* 1991;100:1007–1011.

40. Palmon SC, Moore LE, Lundberg J, et al. Venous air embolism: a review. *J Clin Anesth* 1997;9:251–257.

41. Chopra SK, Taplin GV. Ventilation-perfusion lung imaging in diaphragmatic paralysis. *South Med J* 1979;72:351–352.

42. Strauss RM, Boyer TD. Hepatic hydrothorax. *Semin Liver Dis* 1997;17:227–232.

43. Nagai S, Izumi T. Bronchiolitis obliterans with organizing pneumonia. *Curr Opin Pulm Med* 1996;2:419–423.

44. Cordier JF, Loire R, Brune J. Idiopathic bronchiolitis obliterans organizing pneumonia. Definition of characteristic clinical profiles in a series of 16 patients. *Chest* 1989;96:999–1004.

45. Ellison E, Lapuerta P, Martin SE. Cytologic features of mycobacterial pleuritis: logistic regression and statistical analysis of a blinded, case-controlled study. *Diagn Cytopathol* 1998; 19:173–176.

46. Soler P, Tazi A, Hance AJ. Pulmonary Langerhans cell granulomatosis. *Curr Opin Pulm Med* 1995;1:406–416.

47. Planken II, Rietveld AP. Rapid onset pulmonary edema (flash edema) in renal artery stenosis. *Neth J Med* 1998;52:116–119.

48. Diamond JR. Flash pulmonary edema and the diagnostic suspicion of occult renal artery stenosis [see comments]. *Am J Kidney Dis* 1993;21:328–330.

49. Mana J, Gomez-Vaquero C, Montero A, et al. Lofgren's syndrome revisited: a study of 186 patients. *Am J Med* 1999; 107:240–245.

50. Suteanu S, Rohan C, Gherasim E, et al. Hypertrophic osteoarthropathy secondary to bronchopulmonary cancer (our experience). *Rom J Intern Med* 1992;30:281–284.

51. Hansen-Flaschen J, Nordberg J. Clubbing and hypertrophic osteoarthropathy. *Clin Chest Med* 1987;8:287–298.

52. Carcassi U. History of hypertrophic osteoarthropathy (HOA). *Clin Exp Rheumatol* 1992;10[Suppl. 7]:3–7.

53. Mark JB. Management of anterior mediastinal tumors. *Semin Surg Oncol* 1990;6:286–290.

54. Kohman LJ. Approach to the diagnosis and staging of mediastinal masses. *Chest* 1993;103:328S–330S.

55. Tikkakoski T, Lohela P, Leppanen M, et al. Ultrasound-guided aspiration biopsy of anterior mediastinal masses. *J Clin Ultrasound* 1991;19:209–214.

56. Nowinski T, Flanagan J, Ruchman M. Lacrimal gland enlargement in familial sarcoidosis. *Ophthalmology* 1983;90: 909–913.
57. Massry GG, Holds JB, Kincaid MC. Sarcoidosis involving the lacrimal gland. *JAMA* 1993;270:508.
58. Al Khouzaie T, Busser JR. A rare cause of dyspnea and arterial hypoxemia [see comments]. *Chest* 1997;112:1681–1682.
59. Sorrentino M, Resnekov L. Patent foramen ovale associated with platypnea and orthodeoxia. *Chest* 1991;100:1157–1158.
60. Seward JB, Hayes DL, Smith HC, et al. Platypnea-orthodeoxia: clinical profile, diagnostic workup, management, and report of seven cases. *Mayo Clin Proc* 1984;59:221–231.
61. Swanson KL, Prakash UB, Stanson AW. Pulmonary arteriovenous fistulas: Mayo Clinic experience, 1982–1997. *Mayo Clin Proc* 1999;74:671–680.
62. Wang HC, Yang PC, Kuo SH, et al. Pulmonary arteriovenous malformation: analysis of 10 cases. *J Formos Med Assoc* 1998;97:97–100.
63. Armstrong P, Wilson AG, Dee P., Hansell DM. *Imaging of diseases of the chest.* Chicago: Yearbook Medical Publishers, 2000.
64. Zeitz HJ. Bronchial asthma, nasal polyps, and aspirin sensitivity: Samter's syndrome. *Clin Chest Med* 1988;9:567–576.
65. Probst L, Stoney P, Jeney E, et al. Nasal polyps, bronchial asthma and aspirin sensitivity. *J Otolaryngol* 1992;21:60–65.
66. Yoshida S, Sakamoto H, Ishizaki Y, et al. Efficacy of leukotriene receptor antagonist in bronchial hyperresponsiveness and hypersensitivity to analgesic in aspirin-intolerant asthma. *Clin Exp Allergy* 2000;30:64–70.
67. Dahlen B, Margolskee DJ, Zetterstrom O, et al. Effect of the leukotriene receptor antagonist MK-0679 on baseline pulmonary function in aspirin sensitive asthmatic subjects [see comments]. *Thorax* 1993;48:1205–1210.
68. Brown SE, Light RW. Pleural effusion associated with pulmonary embolization. *Clin Chest Med* 1985;6:77–81.
69. Rubins JB, Rubins HB. Etiology and prognostic significance of eosinophilic pleural effusions. A prospective study. *Chest* 1996;110:1271–1274.
70. Adelman M, Albelda SM, Gottlieb J, et al. Diagnostic utility of pleural fluid eosinophilia. *Am J Med* 1984;77:915–920.
71. Van Pee D, Vandenplas O, Gillet JB. Metal fume fever. *Eur J Emerg Med* 1998;5:465–466.
72. Gordon T, Fine JM. Metal fume fever. *Occup Med* 1993;8: 504–517.
73. Lynch IJP. Approach to the patient with a solitary pulmonary nodule. In: Kelley WN, Dupont HL, Glick E, et al., eds. *Textbook of internal medicine.* Philadelphia: Lippincott-Raven Publishers, 1997:1951–1953.

74. Sharma OP. Sarcoidosis. In: Kelley WN, Dupont HL, Glick E, et al., eds. *Textbook of internal medicine*. Philadelphia: Lippincott-Raven Publishers, 1997:2018–2021.

75. Newman LS. Significance of the blood beryllium lymphocyte proliferation test. *Environ Health Perspect* 1996;104[Suppl. 5]: 953–956.

76. Rossman MD. Chronic beryllium disease: diagnosis and management. *Environ Health Perspect* 1996;104[Suppl. 5]: 945–947.

77. Aleman C, Alegre J, Armadans L, et al. The value of chest roentgenography in the diagnosis of pneumothorax after thoracentesis. *Am J Med* 1999;107:340–343.

78. Capizzi SA, Prakash UB. Chest roentgenography after outpatient thoracentesis. *Mayo Clin Proc* 1998;73:948–950.

RENAL

1. Once glomerulonephritis has been established, one step in determining the specific cause is to measure the **serum complement** level. The differential of hypocomplementemic glomerulonephritis includes poststreptococcal glomerulonephritis, endocarditis, cryoglobulinemia, membranoproliferative glomerulonephritis, shunt nephritis, cholesterol emboli syndrome, and systemic lupus erythematosus (SLE). The differential of normocomplementemic glomerulonephritis includes Wegener granulomatosis, Goodpasture syndrome, microscopic polyarteritis nodosa, and Henoch-Schönlein purpura (1).

2. Only a few diseases lead to chronic renal failure while maintaining **normal to large kidney size**. Included in this list are diabetes mellitus (DM), amyloidosis, human immunodeficiency virus-associated nephropathy (HIVAN), and other infiltrative diseases of the kidney (e.g., lymphoma). Polycystic kidney disease (PKD) causes markedly enlarged kidneys (2–4).

3. In acute renal failure, the creatinine level typically rises by no more than 1.5 mg/dl/day. Any patient who has a more rapid rise in creatinine may have **rhabdomyolysis** with release of large amounts of creatinine from skeletal muscle (5).

4. **Bartter syndrome** is considered in the differential diagnosis of metabolic alkalosis, hypokalemia, and hypomagnesemia. Most cases are diagnosed in childhood, with predominant symptoms of polyuria and weakness secondary to hypokalemia. Growth and mental retardation occur in some cases. One way

of differentiating Bartter syndrome from Cushing syndrome, primary hyperaldosteronism (Conn syndrome), and Liddle syndrome is that patients with Bartter syndrome have normal blood pressure as opposed to the latter three which may present with elevations in blood pressure (6,7).

5. **Alport syndrome** (hereditary nephritis) should be considered in young men who present with recurrent glomerular hematuria, proteinuria, renal insufficiency, sensorineural hearing loss, and eye abnormalities (e.g., anterior lenticonus). This syndrome should be differentiated from other forms of glomerular hematuria, such as thin basement membrane disease, which causes hematuria in the absence of renal insufficiency, and IgA nephropathy, which causes recurrent hematuria and renal insufficiency, but lacks the extra renal manifestations of Alport syndrome (e.g., hearing and eye changes). A renal biopsy may be necessary to differentiate Alport syndrome from IgA nephropathy. It is currently possible to perform skin biopsy and test for Alport syndrome (8,9).

6. When a patient presents with hyponatremia it is usually fairly straightforward to assess whether the condition arises from hypervolemic hyponatremia (presence of pitting edema, pulmonary rales, ascites). It can sometimes be more difficult to differentiate hypovolemic hyponatremia from euvolemic hyponatremia. One useful laboratory test that may discriminate between the two is a **serum uric acid** level that is typically elevated in hypovolemic hyponatremia and decreased (less than 4 mg/dl) in the syndrome of inappropriate antidiuretic hormone secretion (10).

7. **Bartter syndrome** and **Gitelman syndrome** are two disorders that need to be distinguished from each other because their clinical presentations may be similar. Both diseases can lead to renal wasting of potassium and magnesium. Bartter syndrome is typically diagnosed in childhood with growth and mental retardation—but not always. These patients have metabolic alkalosis, hypokalemia, hypomagne-

semia, hyperreninemia, and hyperaldosteronism with normotension. The normal blood pressure is important because most patients with hyperaldosteronism are hypertensive. Gitelman syndrome manifests as hypomagnesemia (more severe than Bartter syndrome), hypokalemia, with low-normal blood pressure. One helpful way to distinguish the two is to remember that Bartter syndrome has the metabolic abnormalities of a loop diuretic: hypokalemia, hypomagnesemia, and hypercalciuria. Gitelman syndrome can be compared to thiazide diuretic therapy: hypomagnesemia, hypokalemia, and hypocalciuria (11,12).

8. Ingestion of certain forms of **licorice** can result in a condition that resembles primary aldosteronism. Glycyrrhizic acid is the component in licorice that causes sodium retention, expansion of extracellular fluid volume, hypertension, and hypokalemia. The compound inhibits 11-β hydroxysteroid dehydrogenase and does not allow cortisol degradation to cortisone. In these cases, excess cortisol acts as a mineral corticoid in principal cells where sodium is reabsorbed and potassium is excreted (13,14).

9. The diagnosis of **Liddle syndrome** should be considered in patients with hypertension and hypokalemia, in the absence of potassium wasting diuretics, no evidence of Cushing syndrome, and **low levels** of renin and aldosterone. The defect is in the epithelial sodium channel in principal cells, leading to excess sodium reabsorption in the renal tubule that is linked to potassium excretion (6,15).

10. **Milk-alkali syndrome** should be considered in the differential diagnosis of hypercalcemia. The tetrad of hypercalcemia, renal insufficiency, chloride responsive metabolic alkalosis, and a history of calcium and alkali ingestion solidifies this diagnosis (16).

11. Chronic nonsteroidal inflammatory drug (NSAID) use can cause nephrotic syndrome and renal insufficiency. **Minimal change disease** is the classic glomerular pathology, but membranous nephropathy can be seen (17,18).

12. Uric acid kidney stones are **radiolucent** and, therefore, cannot be detected on plain films (19).

13. A patient who presents with constipation, nephrocalcinosis, and a 12-lead electrocardiogram (ECG) that demonstrates a shortened QT interval likely has acute symptomatic **hypercalcemia** (20).

14. Two disease entities should be considered in a patient with underlying coronary artery disease who develops acute renal failure after angiography: (a) **radiocontrast-induced renal failure** or (b) **atheroembolic disease** (cholesterol emboli syndrome). Contrast nephropathy occurs in patients with underlying renal insufficiency (Cr >1.5 mg/dl), diabetic nephropathy, or congestive heart failure. The onset of renal failure occurs soon after the contrast is administered and full recovery within 1 to 3 weeks is the rule in most cases. Cholesterol emboli syndrome occurs after vascular procedures (e.g., angiography) or initiation of anticoagulation with coumadin. It presents with evidence of embolic phenomenon such as blue toes or Hollenhorst plaques (cholesterol emboli in retinal arterioles), dermatologic findings (livedo reticularis), eosinophilia or eosinophiluria, hypocomplementemia, and renal failure. The prognosis is worse for atheroembolic disease than for radiocontrast-induced nephropathy (21–23).

15. The diagnosis of **familial hypocalciuric hypercalcemia (FHH)** should be excluded with a 24-hour urine calcium collection and family history before making the definitive diagnosis of primary hyperparathyroidism. This is important because no benefit is seen to parathyroidectomy in a patient with FHH (24).

16. **Sjögren syndrome**, one of the most common systemic diseases leading to distal renal tubular acidosis (RTA) in adults, should be suspected in a patient who presents with hypokalemia and a nonanion-gap acidosis (25).

17. **Renal tubular acidosis** should be considered in patients who present with nonanion-gap acidosis.

The diagnosis of proximal or distal RTA is likely in the presence of hypokalemia and the absence of diarrhea. Distal RTA is more likely than proximal if the urine pH is consistently alkaline. The most likely causes of distal RTA in an adult are autoimmune (Sjögren syndrome, rheumatoid arthritis), hypercalciuria, and chemotherapy with ifosfamide (26,27).

18. **Polyuria** can be defined by urine output greater than 3 L/day. In the absence of uncontrolled DM leading to an osmotic diuresis, three main disorders cause polyuria, all of which are associated with urine osmolality less than 250 mOsm/kg: primary polydipsia, central diabetes insipidus (DI), and nephrogenic DI. Causes of central DI include neurosurgery, autoimmune diseases, trauma, primary and metastatic tumors, and infiltrative diseases (e.g., sarcoidosis and histiocytosis X). The major causes of nephrogenic DI in adults are chronic lithium use and hypercalcemia (28–32).

19. **Renovascular hypertension** is one of the more common causes of secondary hypertension, especially moderate to severe hypertension. A diagnosis of renal artery stenosis should be pursued in patients whose creatinine level rises after institution of an angiotensin converting enzyme inhibitor; in patients greater than 50 years of age who develop difficult-to-control hypertension in the setting of diffuse atherosclerotic disease (especially with a unilateral abdominal bruit); moderate to severe hypertension and asymmetrically sized kidneys; and hypertension and flash pulmonary edema (33).

20. In a patient with an active urinary sediment with red blood cell casts, renal failure, and normal complement level, it is prudent to order antiglomerular basement membrane antibodies. This is an important step because the treatment of anti-glomerular basement membrane disease or **Goodpasture syndrome** (associated pulmonary hemorrhage) is different from that for the vasculitides, consisting of emergent plasma

exchange in addition to steroid and cytotoxic therapy. It has been shown that one of the most important prognostic factors is the creatinine level before the institution of therapy. Patients with creatinine values greater than 5 to 6 mg/dl typically do not recover their renal function (34).

21. Substantial differential diagnosis exists for **hypercalcemia**, but the most common cause of hypercalcemia in the outpatient setting is primary hyperparathyroidism. In an inpatient setting, the most common cause of symptomatic hypercalcemia is malignancy. It is important to rule out other less common causes of hypercalcemia (e.g., medications, endocrinopathies, granulomatous diseases, milk-alkali syndrome, and FHH) (35,36).

22. Rapidly progressive renal failure with anemia and a markedly elevated lactate dehydrogenase should raise suspicion for the **hemolytic-uremic syndrome** (37).

23. **PKD** is one of the few causes of chronic renal failure that maintains a normal hematocrit. Chronic renal failure with a preserved hematocrit should raise the specter of PKD (38,39).

24. A patient with **type I DM** who develops significant proteinuria in the absence of diabetic retinopathy suggests that the proteinuria may not be caused by diabetes. In short, in type I DM, retinopathy should precede nephropathy (40,41).

25. Macroglossia and nephrotic syndrome is **amyloidosis** until proved otherwise (42).

26. Renal insufficiency secondary to **postrenal obstruction** can occur with increased urine output, normal urine output, or decreased urine output. Normal urine output does not rule out postrenal obstruction as a cause for renal failure (43).

27. **Rhabdomyolysis** should be considered in patients with acute renal failure who have a heme-positive urinalysis in the absence of red blood cells. This is a clue to the presence of pigment nephropathy (myoglobin or hemoglobin) (44,45).

28. Acute renal failure in the presence of marked hyperuricemia, hyperkalemia, hyperphosphatemia, and hypocalcemia suggests **tumor lysis syndrome (TLS)** as the underlying cause. TLS classically occurs days following chemotherapy for treatment of rapidly growing tumors (46).

29. **Pulmonary hemorrhage** secondary to SLE usually occurs in the setting of lupus nephritis (47).

30. **Scleroderma renal crisis** should be considered in patients (women more commonly than men) who develop rapidly progressive renal failure in the setting of malignant hypertension and microangiopathic hemolytic anemia. Angiotensin converting enzyme inhibitors have been vital to the treatment of scleroderma renal crisis and have been shown to improve survival. Most of these patients who develop scleroderma renal crisis carry the preexisting diagnosis of scleroderma (48).

31. In a patient with acute renal failure, the triad of fever, skin rash, and eosinophilia points toward the diagnosis of **acute interstitial nephritis (AIN)**. Only a few patients present with this triad. Acute renal failure following drug therapy, infections, and collagen vascular diseases should raise the possibility of AIN. The most common drugs implicated in AIN are β-lactam antibiotics (penicillin, cephalosporins), NSAIDS, and sulfa-containing medications. SLE and Sjögren syndrome are collagen-vascular diseases implicated. Sarcoidosis, another cause of AIN, should be considered in patients with chronic dyspnea, cough, adenopathy, and renal insufficiency. Eosinophiluria, when seen in AIN, makes drug-induced AIN more likely (10,49–51).

32. **Indinavir**, one of the prototypical protease inhibitors, causes both indinavir crystal nephrolithiasis as well as AIN in patients infected with HIV (52,53).

33. **HIVAN** can be differentiated from **heroin-induced nephropathy** by a number of methods: the time course to end-stage renal disease is different, with HIVAN occurring over several weeks to months and heroin nephropathy occurring over several years.

Ultrasound imaging classically demonstrates normal to enlarged kidneys with HIVAN and reduced kidney size with heroin nephropathy (54).

34. The **urine anion-gap** may help differentiate diarrhea and a distal RTA. Patients with diarrhea have normal ability to excrete acid, which is excreted primarily as NH_4Cl. The urine ion gap ($U_{NA} + U_K - U_{CL}$) is negative. Patients with distal RTA are unable to excrete acid in urine properly, leading to decreased urine NH_4Cl. The urine anion gap is positive. The urine anion gap should be reserved for nonanion gap acidosis with urine sodium greater than 25 mEq/L (26).

35. The combination of rapidly progressive glomerulonephritis, pulmonary alveolar hemorrhage, positive pANCA, and lack of upper respiratory tract involvement (sinusitis, otitis media, mastoiditis, nasal septal perforation) is consistent with the diagnosis of **microscopic polyangiitis**. The lack of upper respiratory tract involvement and granulomas on biopsy makes Wegener granulomatosis less likely, whereas glomerulonephritis makes classic polyarteritis nodosa unlikely. A positive pANCA is more common with microscopic polyangiitis than with Wegener granulomatosis (55).

36. Consider the diagnosis of multiple myeloma in a patient who presents with anemia, bone pain, hypokalemia, hypophosphatemia, glycosuria (with a normal serum glucose level), and nonanion gap metabolic acidosis. This **Fanconi-like syndrome**, as part of a proximal renal tubular acidosis, can be a rare presentation of multiple myeloma in an adult. The bone pain may be secondary to myeloma-induced osteolytic lesions or secondary to chronic hypophosphatemic osteomalacia (56).

37. The triad of chronic renal failure, secondary hyperparathyroidism, and cutaneous necrotic ulceration points to a diagnosis of systemic **calciphylaxis**. This disorder is characterized clinically by epidermal ulceration, dermal necrosis, and chronic calcifying septal panniculitis in the setting of chronic renal

failure (57,58). More recent reports demonstrate secondary hyperparathyroidism is not necessary for calciphylaxis (59).

38. The most common cause of kidney disease in patients with underlying hepatitis C virus (HCV) is **membrano-proliferative glomerulonephritis** (60).

39. Patients with SLE who have antibodies to double-stranded DNA are more likely to present with **lupus nephritis** than patients who are ds-DNA negative (61).

40. The tetrad of hypocomplementemic glomerulonephri-tis, arthralgias, peripheral neuropathy, and Raynaud phenomenon is concerning for **mixed cryoglobu-linemia** (type II). C4 is typically reduced more com-monly than C3 and rheumatoid factor is often positive. A strong correlation is found between essential mixed cryoglobulinemia and HCV infection (62–64).

41. **Nephrotoxicity** associated with aminoglycoside is increased with concomitant vancomycin adminis-tration (65).

42. **Poststreptococcal glomerulonephritis (PSGN)** typ-ically occurs 7 to 14 days after an upper respiratory infection with *Streptococcus pyogenes*. PSGN is char-acterized by acute renal failure, hematuria (Coca-Cola urine), proteinuria, edema, and, at times, hyperten-sion. Most (90%) cases are in children and most cases are self-limited. PSGN can cause persistent hyper-tension and chronic renal insufficiency in adults. C3 is characteristically depressed to a greater degree than C4 (66).

43. **Emphysematous pyelonephritis (EP)** is a necro-tizing infection of the renal parenchyma caused by gas-forming organisms, most commonly *Escherichia coli*. The initial clinical features consist of flank pain, fever, and urinalysis consistent with bacterial infec-tion. EP most commonly affects patients with under-lying DM and carries a high mortality rate. Antibiotic therapy alone is usually ineffective and percutaneous drainage, nephrectomy, or both are often necessary. This diagnosis should be considered in toxic patients

with underlying DM who present with pyelonephritis unresponsive to antibiotics. CT scan is the imaging test of choice to evaluate for gas in the kidney (67,68).

44. Patients with chronically infected ventriculoatrial shunts can develop an **immune complex glomeru-lonephritis (shunt nephritis)** characterized by renal insufficiency, hematuria, proteinuria, and hypocomplementemia. Early antibiotic therapy and removal of the infected shunt are imperative to prevent irreversible renal failure (69).

45. **Aluminum toxicity** should be considered in patients in chronic renal failure who are treated with aluminum-based phosphate binders to reduce hyperphosphatemia. Clinical features of chronic aluminum toxicity include dementia of unknown origin, osteomalacia, and anemia refractory to erythropoietin. Chronic sucralfate therapy may also lead to aluminum toxicity (70–72).

46. Although much more frequent in children, hematuria, renal insufficiency, large joint lower extremity arthritis, and palpable purpura in adults should prompt an investigation for **Henoch-Schönlein purpura**, a small vessel systemic vasculitis. Skin biopsy should demonstrate leukocytoclastic vasculitis with IgA deposition on immunofluorescence staining (73,74).

47. The tetrad of obtundation, anion gap metabolic acidosis, osmolar gap, and calcium oxalate crystals in the urine makes **ethylene glycol intoxication** a leading diagnosis. Patients who present with a severe anion-gap acidosis and osmolar gap of unknown cause should have their urine analyzed for calcium oxalate crystals, a breakdown product of ethylene glycol (75,76).

REFERENCES

1. Madaio MP, Harrington JT. Current concepts. The diagnosis of acute glomerulonephritis. *N Engl J Med* 1983;309:1299–1302.
2. Obrador GT, Price B, O'Meara Y, et al. Acute renal failure due to lymphomatous infiltration of the kidneys. *J Am Soc Nephrol* 1997;8:1348–1354.

3. Derchi LE, Martinoli C, Saffioti S, et al. Ultrasonographic imaging and Doppler analysis of renal changes in non-insulin-dependent diabetes mellitus. *Acad Radiol* 1994;1:100–105.

4. Hiraoka M, Hori C, Tsuchida S, et al. Ultrasonographic findings of acute tubulointerstitial nephritis. *Am J Nephrol* 1996; 16:154–158.

5. Woodrow G, Brownjohn AM, Turney JH. The clinical and biochemical features of acute renal failure due to rhabdomyolysis. *Ren Fail* 1995;17:467–474.

6. Scheinman SJ, Guay-Woodford LM, Thakker RV, et al. Genetic disorders of renal electrolyte transport. *N Engl J Med* 1999;340:1177–1187.

7. Bartholow C, Whittier FC, Rutecki GW. Hypokalemia and metabolic alkalosis: algorithms for combined clinical problem solving. *Compr Ther* 2000;26:114–120.

8. Jais JP, Knebelmann B, Giatras I, et al. X-linked Alport syndrome: natural history in 195 families and genotype-phenotype correlations in males. *J Am Soc Nephrol* 2000;11:649–657.

9. Frasca GM, Onetti-Muda A, Renieri A. Thin glomerular basement membrane disease. *J Nephrol* 2000;13:15–19.

10. Michel DM, Kelly CJ. Acute interstitial nephritis. *J Am Soc Nephrol* 1998;9:506–515.

11. Dell KM, Guay-Woodford LM. Inherited tubular transport disorders. *Semin Nephrol* 1999;19:364–373.

12. Singh PJ, Nash JL, Santella RN, et al. Gitelman's syndrome: report of a 19-year-old woman with intractable hypomagnesemia and hypokalemia, and a review of the syndrome. *S D J Med* 1999;52:377–380.

13. de Klerk GJ, Nieuwenhuis MG, Beutler JJ. Hypokalaemia and hypertension associated with use of liquorice flavoured chewing gum. *BMJ* 1997;314:731–732.

14. Heikens J, Fliers E, Endert E, et al. Liquorice-induced hypertension—a new understanding of an old disease: case report and brief review. *Neth J Med* 1995;47:230–234.

15. Botero-Velez M, Curtis JJ, Warnock DG. Brief report: Liddle's syndrome revisited—a disorder of sodium reabsorption in the distal tubule. *Arch Intern Med* 1993;153:1005–1010.

16. George S, Clark JD. Milk alkali syndrome—an unusual syndrome causing an unusual complication. *Postgrad Med J* 2000;76:422–424.

17. Rotellar JA, Garcia RC, Martinez VA, et al. Minimal-change glomerulopathy associated with diclofenac: response to prednisone [Letter, comment]. *Am J Kidney Dis* 1089;14:530–531.

18. Marasco WA, Gikas PW, Azziz-Baumgartner R, et al. Ibuprofen-associated renal dysfunction. Pathophysiologic mechanisms of acute renal failure, hyperkalemia, tubular

necrosis, and proteinuria. *Arch Intern Med* 1987;147: 2107–2116.

19. Halabe A, Sperling O. Uric acid nephrolithiasis. *Miner Electrolyte Metab* 1994;20:424–431.
20. Ahmed R, Hashiba K. Reliability of QT intervals as indicators of clinical hypercalcemia. *Clin Cardiol* 1988;11:395–400.
21. Solomon R. Radiocontrast-induced nephropathy. *Semin Nephrol* 1998;18:551–557.
22. Solomon R, Werner C, Mann D, et al. Effects of saline, mannitol, and furosemide to prevent acute decreases in renal function induced by radiocontrast agents [see comments]. *N Engl J Med* 1994;331:1416–1420.
23. Thadhani RI, Camargo CA, Jr., Xavier RJ, et al. Atheroembolic renal failure after invasive procedures. Natural history based on 52 histologically proven cases. *Medicine (Baltimore)* 1995;74:350–358.
24. Marx SJ, Stock JL, Attie MF, et al. Familial hypocalciuric hypercalcemia: recognition among patients referred after unsuccessful parathyroid exploration. *Ann Intern Med* 1980; 92:351–356.
25. Siamopoulos KC, Elisaf M, Drosos AA, et al. Renal tubular acidosis in primary Sjogren's syndrome. *Clin Rheumatol* 1992;11:226–230.
26. Battle DC, Hizon M, Cohen E, et al. The use of the urinary anion gap in the diagnosis of hyperchloremic metabolic acidosis. *N Engl J Med* 1988;318:594–599.
27. Smulders YM, Frissen PH, Slaats EH, et al. Renal tubular acidosis. Pathophysiology and diagnosis. *Arch Intern Med* 1996;156:1629–1636.
28. Adam P. Evaluation and management of diabetes insipidus. *Am Fam Physician* 1997;55:2146–2153.
29. Differential diagnosis of polyuria [Letter]. *N Engl J Med* 1982; 307:125–126.
30. Knoers NV, Monnens LL. Nephrogenic diabetes insipidus. *Semin Nephrol* 1999;19:344–352.
31. Singer IJ, Oster R, Fishman LM. The management of diabetes insipidus in adults. *Arch Intern Med* 1997;157:1293–1301.
32. Robinson AG, Verbalis JG. Diabetes insipidus. *Curr Ther Endocrinol Metab* 1997;6:1–7.
33. Case records of the Massachusetts General Hospital. Weekly Clinicopathological Exercises. Case 11—1996. A 69-year-old man with progressive renal failure and the abrupt onset of dyspnea [clinical conference] [see comments]. *N Engl J Med* 1996;334:973–979.
34. Case records of the Massachusetts General Hospital. Weekly clinicopathological exercises. Case 52—1993. A

17-year-old girl with massive hemoptysis and acute oliguric renal failure [clinical conference]. *N Engl J Med* 1993;329: 2019–2026.

35. Mow BM, Adlakha A, Rosenow EC, III. 64-year-old man with polyuria and polydipsia. *JAMA* 1982;247:75–80.

36. Case records of the Massachusetts General Hospital. Weekly clinicopathological exercises. Case 26—1982. Hypercalcemia 10 months after chemotherapy for lymphoma. *N Engl J Med* 1982;307:41–49.

37. Thompson CE, Damon LE, Ries CA, et al. Thrombotic microangiopathies in the 1980s: clinical features, response to treatment, and the impact of the human immunodeficiency virus epidemic. *Blood* 1992;80:1890–1895.

38. Rotellar C, Gelfand MC. Polycystic kidneys do maintain good endocrine function. *Med Hypotheses* 1989;30:61–64.

39. Gabow PA. Autosomal dominant polycystic kidney disease. *N Engl J Med* 1993;329:332–342.

40. Wirta O, Pasternack A, Mustonen J, et al. Retinopathy is independently related to microalbuminuria in type 2 diabetes mellitus. *Clin Nephrol* 1999;51:329–334.

41. Campos-Pastor MM, Escobar-Jimenez F, Mezquita P, et al. Factors associated with microalbuminuria in type 1 diabetes mellitus: a cross-sectional study. *Diabetes Res Clin Pract* 2000;48:43–49.

42. Kyle RA, Bayrd ED. Amyloidosis: review of 236 cases. *Medicine (Baltimore)* 1975;54:271–299.

43. Dornfeld L, Narins RG. Pre- and postoperative renal failure. *Urol Clin North Am* 1976;3:363–377.

44. Vanholder R, Sever MS, Erek E, et al. Rhabdomyolysis. *J Am Soc Nephrol* 2000;11:1553–1561.

45. Visweswaran P, Guntupalli J. Rhabdomyolysis. *Crit Care Clin* 1999;15:415–428, ix–x.

46. Arrambide K, Toto RD. Tumor lysis syndrome. *Semin Nephrol* 1993;13:273–280.

47. Zamora MR, Warner ML, Tuder R, et al. Diffuse alveolar hemorrhage and systemic lupus erythematosus. Clinical presentation, histology, survival, and outcome. *Medicine (Baltimore)* 1997;76:192–202.

48. Steen VD. Scleroderma renal crisis. *Rheum Dis Clin North Am* 1996;22:861–878.

49. Reddy S, Salant DJ. Treatment of acute interstitial nephritis. *Ren Fail* 1998;20:829–838.

50. Alexopoulos E. Drug-induced acute interstitial nephritis. *Ren Fail* 1998;20:809–819.

51. Koselj M, Kveder R, Bren AF, et al. Acute renal failure in patients with drug-induced acute interstitial nephritis. *Ren Fail* 1993;15:69–72.

52. Jaradat M, Phillips C, Yum MN, et al. Acute tubulointerstitial nephritis attributable to indinavir therapy. *Am J Kidney Dis* 2000;35:E16.
53. Kohan AD, Armenakas NA, Fracchia JA. Indinavir urolithiasis: an emerging cause of renal colic in patients with human immunodeficiency virus. *J Urol* 1999;161:1765–1768.
54. D'Agati V, Appel GB. Renal pathology of human immunodeficiency virus infection. *Semin Nephrol* 1998;18:406–421.
55. Case records of the Massachusetts General Hospital. Weekly clinicopathological exercises. Case 52—1993. A 17 year-old girl with massive hemoptysis and acute oliguric renal failure [clinical conference]. *N Engl J Med* 1993;329:2019–2026.
56. Gregory MJ, Schwartz GJ. Diagnosis and treatment of renal tubular disorders. *Semin Nephrol* 1998;18:317–329.
57. Janigan DT, Hirsch DJ, Klassen GA, et al. Calcified subcutaneous arterioles with infarcts of the subcutis and skin ("calciphylaxis") in chronic renal failure. *Am J Kidney Dis* 2000;35:588–597.
58. Budisavljevic MN, Cheek D, Ploth DW. Calciphylaxis in chronic renal failure. *J Am Soc Nephrol* 1996;7:978–982.
59. Bleyer AJ, Choi M, Igwemezie B, et al. A case control study of proximal calciphylaxis [see comments]. *Am J Kidney Dis* 1998;32:376–383.
60. Jefferson JA, Johnson RJ. Treatment of hepatitis C-associated glomerular disease. *Semin Nephrol* 2000;20:286–292.
61. Cameron JS. Lupus nephritis. *J Am Soc Nephrol* 1999;10:413–424.
62. Sasso EH. The rheumatoid factor response in the etiology of mixed cryoglobulins associated with hepatitis C virus infection. *Ann Med Interne (Paris)* 2000;151:30–40.
63. Lee YH, Ji JD, Yeon JE, et al. Cryoglobulinaemia and rheumatic manifestations in patients with hepatitis C virus infection. *Ann Rheum Dis* 1998;57:728–731.
64. Daoud MS, el Azhary RA, Gibson LE, et al. Chronic hepatitis C, cryoglobulinemia, and cutaneous necrotizing vasculitis. Clinical, pathologic, and immunopathologic study of twelve patients. *J Am Acad Dermatol* 1996;34:219–223.
65. Goetz MB, Sayers J. Nephrotoxicity of vancomycin and aminoglycoside therapy separately and in combination [published erratum appears in *J Antimicrob Chemother* 1993;32(6):925]. *J Antimicrob Chemother* 1993;32:325–334.
66. Richards J. Acute post-streptococcal glomerulonephritis [clinical conference]. *W V Med J* 1991;87:61–65.
67. McDermid KP, Watterson J, van Eeden SF. Emphysematous pyelonephritis: case report and review of the literature. *Diabetes Res Clin Pract* 1999;44:71–75.

68. Shokeir AA, El Azab M, Mohsen T, et al. Emphysematous pyelonephritis: a 15-year experience with 20 cases. *Urology* 1997;49:343–346.

69. Haffner D, Schindera F, Aschoff A, et al. The clinical spectrum of shunt nephritis [see comments]. *Nephrol Dial Transplant* 1997;12:1143–1148.

70. Sherrard DJ. Aluminum and renal osteodystrophy. *Semin Nephrol* 1986;6:5–11.

71. Yaqoob M, Ahmad R, McClelland P, et al. Resistance to recombinant human erythropoietin due to aluminium overload and its reversal by low dose desferrioxamine therapy. *Postgrad Med J* 1993;69:124–128.

72. Hewitt CD, Savory J, Wills MR. Aspects of aluminum toxicity. *Clin Lab Med* 1990;10:403–422.

73. Rai A, Nast C, Adler S. Henoch-Schonlein purpura nephritis. *J Am Soc Nephrol* 1999;10:2637–2644.

74. Rieu P, Noel LH. Henoch-Schonlein nephritis in children and adults. Morphological features and clinicopathological correlations. *Ann Med Interne (Paris)* 1999;150:151–159.

75. Taylor R, Bower J, Salem MM. Acidosis and coma after hemodialysis. *J Am Soc Nephrol* 1997;8:853–856.

76. Goodkin DA, Krishna GG, Narins RG. The role of the anion gap in detecting and managing mixed metabolic acid-base disorders. *Clin Endocrinol Metab* 1984;13:333–349.

RHEUMATOLOGY

1. A negative **rheumatoid factor (RF)** does not exclude the diagnosis of rheumatoid arthritis (RA) because 15% to 25% of patients with RA will remain RF negative (1).

2. The peripheral (appendicular) arthritis associated with **inflammatory bowel disease (IBD)** predominantly affects the large joints of the lower extremity more so than the upper extremity, and typically coincides with IBD flares (2).

3. In **systemic lupus erythematosus (SLE)**, anti–double-stranded DNA and low complements (especially C3) are associated with nephritis (3).

4. The most common rheumatologic disease associated with **secondary Sjögren syndrome** is RA (4).

5. Malar rash, increased photosensitivity, discoid lesions, and oral ulcers comprise the American Rheumatology Association dermatologic criteria for the diagnosis of **SLE**. Scarring alopecia is not one of the criteria, although its presence in the setting of a multisystem disease should heighten suspicion for SLE (5).

6. Historically, **Jaccoud arthropathy** occurs after rheumatic fever, leading to deformities resembling RA. However, it can also be a manifestation of other rheumatic diseases (e.g., SLE and sarcoidosis). This arthritis is deforming but not erosive, in contrast to RA. The deformities of Jaccoud arthropathy and SLE are reducible in contrast to RA (6,7).

7. Osteoarthritis (OA) classically affects weightbearing joints, distal interphalangeal joints, and proximal

interphalangeal joints, as well as the first carpometa-carpal joint. Consider the diagnosis of **hemochro-matosis** in a patient who presents with pain and classic OA findings on plain films (hooklike osteo-phytes on the metacarpal heads) affecting the second and third metacarpophalangeal joints (8).

8. The two most likely drugs to cause **drug-induced lupus** are procainamide and hydralazine. Other drugs less commonly implicated are diltiazem, penicillamine, isoniazid (INH), methyldopa, and chlorpromazine. Clinical features include fever, myalgias or arthralgias, rash, and serositis. In contrast to SLE, drug-induced lupus does not typically involve the kidneys (glomeru-lonephritis), central nervous system (lupus cerebritis), or blood cell lines (cytopenias) (9).

9. Lupus patients have an unusual predisposition to sulfa toxicity (10).

10. Distinguishing **CREST** (*c*alcinosis, *R*aynaud phe-nomenon, *e*sophageal dysmotility, *s*clerodactyly, and *t*elangiectasias) and diffuse scleroderma can be diffi-cult. A useful distinction is that in CREST the skin thickening is limited to the hands and face, whereas in diffuse scleroderma widespread skin thickening progresses from the digits to the trunk (11).

11. **Giant cell arteritis (GCA)** should be considered in pa-tients over 50 years of age who present with new onset headaches and an elevated erythrocyte sedimentation rate . Features that make the diagnosis of GCA more likely include jaw claudication, temporal artery tender-ness, decreased temporal artery pulsation, scalp ten-derness, polymyalgia rheumatica, normocytic anemia, elevated alkaline phosphatase, fevers, and transient loss of vision. The diagnosis is confirmed by demon-strating necrotizing granulomatous inflammation of the temporal artery (or any accessible branch of the great vessels) in the presence of compatible clinical mani-festations. One other helpful clue to the diagnosis of GCA is response to corticosteroids. The diagnosis should be questioned in any patient suspected of GCA who is resistant to corticosteroid therapy (12).

12. **Vasculitis** associated with **RA** is almost never a presenting feature of the disease. RA-associated vasculitis classically occurs in patients with long-standing erosive, nodular RA with high titer RF (13).

13. The triad of degenerative arthritis, urine that turns black on standing, and cartilaginous pigmentation is virtually pathognomonic for **alkaptonuria** (i.e., ochronosis). The ochronotic arthritis is heralded by pain and decreased range of motion of the hips, shoulders, and knees. Often, darkening is seen of the sclera, concha, and helix. Black pigmentation may be seen of the disk space. The compound that builds up in this condition is homogentisic acid (14).

14. A **temporal artery biopsy** performed more than 14 days after initiation of corticosteroid therapy for presumed GCA still demonstrated vasculitis and granulomatous changes. Corticosteroid therapy should not dissuade the use of temporal artery biopsy (15).

15. Magnetic resonance angiography typically does not provide sufficient resolution to demonstrate primary angiitis of the central nervous system. Angiography and brain biopsies are two approaches to confirm this diagnosis (16–18).

16. **Bilateral carpal tunnel syndrome** should raise suspicion for systemic diseases such as diabetes mellitus, hypothyroidism, polyarteritis nodosa (PAN), Churg-Strauss syndrome (CSS), RA, pregnancy, acromegaly, and amyloidosis (19,20).

17. The most common rheumatologic cause of **secondary amyloidosis** is RA. This should be suspected in patients with longstanding RA who develop renal insufficiency with proteinuria (especially nephrotic range) (21).

18. In developing countries, tuberculosis and leprosy are common causes of **secondary amyloidosis**. Consider secondary amyloidosis if an intravenous drug abuser with chronic nonhealing pyogenic infections presents with weight loss and multisystem organ involvement of the kidneys, the gastrointestinal tract, and the heart (21,22).

19. **Classic PAN**, a medium vessel vasculitis, should be suspected in patients who present with the subacute onset of fever, myalgias, weight loss, postprandial abdominal pain, hypertension, renal insufficiency, mononeuritis multiplex, cutaneous ulcers, livedo reticularis, palpable purpura, and testicular pain. An association is seen between hepatitis B infection and PAN. Arteriography may demonstrate multiple aneurysms in different arteries (hepatic and renal) (23).

20. **CSS** is a necrotizing vasculitis characterized by underlying asthma, prominent eosinophilia, and fleeting pulmonary infiltrates. Other features that suggest CSS include mononeuritis multiplex, subcutaneous nodules, cardiomyopathy, and palpable purpura. P-ANCA is positive in most cases (24).

21. **Takayasu arteritis** is a vasculitis that affects patients usually less than 40 years of age. The disease should be suspected in any young adult (women affected more commonly than men) who presents with symptoms of claudication, especially in conjunction with diminished brachial pulses and systemic arterial bruits (subclavian or abdominal aorta). Takayasu arteritis has been referred to as "pulseless disease," and may have a prodrome characterized by fever of unknown origin, weight loss, and malaise. New-onset hypertension may be a clue to the diagnosis because the renal artery is affected in about 50% of patients (25).

22. Consider **disseminated gonococcal infection** with the triad of tenosynovitis, arthralgias, and vesiculopustular skin lesions (26).

23. A patient who presents with a perforated nasal septum and glomerulonephritis has **Wegener granulomatosis (WG)** until proved otherwise. Other causes of perforated nasal septum include midline lethal granuloma, rhinocerebral mucormycosis, syphilis, tuberculosis, and cocaine or heroin inhalation (27).

24. **RA** is associated with several types of lung pathology: Caplan syndrome (pneumoconiosis with rheumatoid nodules), pleural effusions with decreased pleural glu-

cose, interstitial disease, and bronchiolitis obliterans with organizing pneumonia (BOOP). The most common form of RA lung disease is pleural effusion. These pulmonary manifestations of RA are seen more commonly in men (28).

25. Three serious complications of **GCA** are permanent visual loss, cerebral vascular accidents, and thoracic artery aneurysms that have the potential to dissect or rupture (29,30).

26. Four rheumatologic disorders are associated with **aortitis** and **aortic regurgitation**: ankylosing spondylitis, relapsing polychondritis, Reiter syndrome, and RA. Two vasculitic processes that can lead to aortitis are GCA and Takayasu arteritis (31,32).

27. A **saddle nose deformity** in an adult may be an important clue to a systemic disease. WG, relapsing polychondritis, and syphilis are three causes of a saddle nose deformity (33,34).

28. The differential diagnosis of **avascular necrosis** in an adult includes corticosteroid use, alcohol abuse, chronic renal insufficiency, trauma, SLE, and sickle cell disease (35).

29. **Polymyalgia rheumatica (PMR)** can present as a peripheral synovitis that can resemble early, seronegative RA. Commonly affected peripheral joints are knees, wrists, and metacarpophalangeal joints. Of note, the synovitis of PMR responds better to small doses of prednisone than does RA, which may help differentiate these two disease entities (36).

30. **Adult onset Still disease** is a challenging diagnosis because no laboratory abnormality or tissue biopsy finding is pathognomonic. The disease should be suspected in young adults who present with hectic fevers once or twice a day (often at night) and who usually become afebrile at some point during the same 24-hour period. A fleeting salmon-pink maculopapular rash commonly located on the trunk is the telltale sign of this disease and is frequently coincident with the fever

spikes. A mild arthritis is often present and most commonly affects the knees and wrists. The ankles, shoulders, and proximal interphalangeal joints are affected in 50% of cases. Radiographically, nonerosive narrowing of the carpometacarpal joints is most common. Anemia, thrombocytosis, leukocytosis, elevated aminotransferases, elevated ferritin (often >3000 μg/L), hepatosplenomegaly, lymphadenopathy, and sore throat are other manifestations that point toward this elusive diagnosis (37).

31. In patients with underlying **polymyositis** who are treated with glucocorticoids and have increased muscle weakness, it can be challenging to differentiate exacerbations of the polymyositis from **corticosteroid myopathy**. Serial creatinine phosphokinase levels can help differentiate the two, because an exacerbation of polymyositis should be accompanied by increases in creatine phosphokinase, whereas corticosteroid myopathy is not (38).

32. **Behçet syndrome** should be considered in the differential diagnosis for any young adult who presents with recurrent painful oral (>3 episodes in 1 year) or genital ulcers. Other major criteria for diagnosis include aseptic meningitis, uveitis, pathergy (pustulosis following skin injury), cutaneous manifestations (acneiform lesions, erythema nodosumlike lesions, purpura, papulopustular lesions, pyoderma gangrenosum-type ulcers). IBD should be excluded before rendering a diagnosis of Behçet syndrome because of similar clinical features. One potentially fatal complication of this disease is a pulmonary artery-bronchus fistula (virtually pathognomonic of Behçet syndrome) which can present as massive hemoptysis. Diagnosis is made by pulmonary angiogram (39).

33. Consider the diagnosis of **Felty syndrome** in a patient with longstanding RA who presents with increasing frequency of infections. This syndrome is the triad of RA, splenomegaly, and neutropenia. These patients typically have high titers of RF and erosive, nodular RA (40).

34. Intense attacks of **Raynaud phenomenon (RP)** or an initial attack that has its onset after the age of 40 should raise suspicion for an underlying systemic disease. The most common connective tissue disease associated with RP is scleroderma (>90% of patients with scleroderma have RP). Other connective tissue diseases associated with RP are polymyositis, dermatomyositis (DM), Sjögren syndrome, SLE, systemic vasculitis, and mixed connective tissue disease. Dilated nailbed capillary loops and loss of normal capillaries in the nailfold point toward three diagnoses: scleroderma, DM, and SLE. Nailbed capillary dropout makes scleroderma the most likely diagnosis (41–43).

35. A patient who presents with **septic monoarthritis** and synovial fluid cultures growing *Staphylococcus aureus*, group C or G streptococci, or enterococci, with no obvious source may have underlying endocarditis, especially if an intravenous drug abuser (44,45).

36. **Impaired chest expansion** (normally >4 to 5 cm with deep inspiration) may be an early clue to the diagnosis of ankylosing spondylitis. This is a physical examination finding seen in young men who present with inflammatory low back or buttock pain (pain improves with exercise) (46).

37. Vasculitis causing pulmonary hemorrhage most commonly occurs **in antineutrophil cytoplasmic antibody (ANCA)-associated disease**, which includes WG and microscopic polyangiitis (MPA). WG should be suspected in patients with upper respiratory tract abnormalities (sinusitis, epistaxis, otitis media, saddle-nose deformity, subglottic stenosis), lower respiratory tract abnormalities (nodules, cavitary lesions, diffuse pulmonary infiltrates connoting alveolar hemorrhage), and renal abnormalities (focal segmental glomerulonephritis). Some patients have a limited form of disease with only upper and lower respiratory tract involvement. MPA can resemble WG; MPA, however, does not produce granulomatous inflammation and is associated with p-ANCA, whereas WG is usually associated with c-ANCA (47,48).

38. **Calcium pyrophosphate dihydrate disease (CPPD)** is most commonly asymptomatic in adults, but can mimic other rheumatologic diseases such as gout (pseudogout), RA (pseudo-RA), Charcot joint, and OA. When symptomatic, CPPD most commonly presents as a "goutylike attack" with pain, redness, and swelling of a single joint. The knee and wrist are to CPPD what the great toe and ankle are to gout–the most common sites of disease. Joint aspirate and fluid analysis can differentiate these two diseases. Secondary causes of CPPD include hemochromatosis, Wilson disease, hyperparathyroidism, hypothyroidism, hypomagnesemia, familial hypocalciuric hypercalcemia, and ochronosis (49).

39. **Hidradenitis suppurativa** has been associated with spondyloarthropathy and should be considered in the differential diagnosis of inflammatory low back pain (50).

40. The diagnosis of **acute rheumatic fever (ARF)** can be challenging, especially in the absence of carditis. Migratory polyarthritis in a younger patient should invoke the possibility of ARF. Although not considered a major criterion for diagnosis, serology can be sent for antibodies against the group A streptococcal organism. Subcutaneous nodules, similar to those seen in RA, located around the olecranon process comprise a major criterion for ARF (51).

41. **Enthesopathy**, which is inflammation of the ligament or tendon at the point where it inserts into bone, presents clinically as pain at the Achilles tendon and in the hindfoot (plantar fasciitis). The differential diagnosis includes the seronegative spondyloarthropathies: Reiter syndrome, ankylosing spondylitis, psoriatic arthritis, and arthritis associated with IBD (52).

42. Dermatomyositis and polymyositis are both associated with interstitial lung disease. A subset of these patients are anti-Jo-1 (**tRNA-histidyl transferase**) positive. In addition to interstitial lung disease, this subset classically presents with fever, RP, arthritis, and mechanic hands. The patients who have the

myositis and interstitial lung disease tend not to develop the malignancies associated with myositis (e.g., ovarian cancer) (53,54).

43. **Psoriatic arthritis (PA)** can present with various clinical manifestations: asymmetric oligoarthritis, symmetric polyarthritis (RA-like), DIPitis (inflammation of the distal interphalangeal joints), sacroiliitis, and arthritis mutilans (which can cause destruction out of proportion to pain). The symmetric polyarthritis and asymmetric oligoarthritis are the most common forms of PA, whereas DIPitis (inflammation of the distal interphalangeal joints; the rarest form of PA) is associated with nail pitting (55,56).

44. The diagnosis of **fibromyalgia** should be challenged in a patient whose symptoms involve the hands or whose physical examination demonstrates objective joint pathology (red-hot swollen joint) (57).

45. Auscultate for bruits in a young woman who presents with systemic hypertension and decreased radial pulses. The finding of multiple bruits suggests **Takayasu arteritis** (58).

46. **Spondylitis** associated with IBD typically progresses, independently of IBD flares (59).

47. The most common **extraarticular** manifestation of ankylosing spondylitis is anterior uveitis (60).

48. The arthritis of psoriasis is generally **less tender** than that of RA (56).

49. The severity of **psoriatic arthritis** does not necessarily correlate with the severity of the skin disease. It is important to examine the patient's skin in its entirety, because occasionally the only clinical signs of psoriasis can be subtle nail pitting, an inconspicuous intragluteal plaque, a single patch behind the ears, or an isolated scalp lesion (61).

50. **Mononeuritis multiplex** in the absence of diabetes and multiple compression injuries indicates the patient has vasculitis. PAN and WG are the most common forms of vasculitis associated with mononeuritis multiplex (62).

51. In trying to differentiate PAN from WG, new onset **hypertension** suggests PAN (23).

52. Strong suspicion of **GCA** should prompt treatment first (steroids) followed by biopsy. Intravenous steroids should be used if the patient has had visual loss (63).

53. A patient with RA who has only one active joint should be suspected of having **septic arthritis** (64).

54. **Dermatomyositis** in adults can be associated with malignancy, especially ovarian cancer in women (65).

55. The most common cause of death in **SLE** is infection. Infection can mimic or be superimposed upon active SLE (66).

56. **Gout** can be the first manifestation of systemic disease, including polycythemia vera (67,68).

57. Recurrent palpable purpura suggests **cryoglobulinemia**. The most common cause in the urban setting is hepatitis C infection (69).

REFERENCES

1. Shmerling RH, Delbanco TL. How useful is the rheumatoid factor? An analysis of sensitivity, specificity, and predictive value [see comments]. *Arch Intern Med* 1992;152:2417–2420.
2. Gravallese EM, Kantrowitz FG. Arthritic manifestations of inflammatory bowel disease. *Am J Gastroenterol* 1988;83:703–709.
3. Schur PH, Sandson J. Immunologic factors and clinical activity in systemic lupus erythematosus. *N Engl J Med* 1968;278:533–538.
4. Moutsopoulos HM, Chused TM, Mann DL, et al. Sjogren's syndrome (Sicca syndrome): current issues. *Ann Intern Med* 1980;92:212–226.
5. Hochberg MC. Updating the American College of Rheumatology revised criteria for the classification of systemic lupus erythematosus [Letter] [see comments]. *Arthritis Rheum* 1997; 40:1725.
6. van Vugt RM, Derksen RH, Kater L, et al. Deforming arthropathy or lupus and rhupus hands in systemic lupus erythematosus. *Ann Rheum Dis* 1998;57:540–544.
7. Ignaczak T, Espinoza LR, Kantor OS, et al. Jaccoud arthritis. *Arch Intern Med* 1975;135:577–579.

8. Schumacher HR, Jr. Arthropathy in hemochromatosis. *Hosp Pract (Off Ed)* 1998;33:81–90, 93.

9. Price EJ, Venables PJ. Drug-induced lupus. *Drug Saf* 1995; 12:283–290.

10. Petri M, Allbritton J. Antibiotic allergy in systemic lupus erythematosus: a case-control study [see comments]. *J Rheumatol* 1992;19:265–269.

11. Steen VD. Clinical manifestations of systemic sclerosis. *Semin Cutan Med Surg* 1998;17:48–54.

12. Hoffman GS. Vasculitis. In: Klippel JH, Weyand CM, Wortman RL, eds. *Primer on the rheumatic diseases.* Atlanta: Arthritis Foundation, 1997:294–295.

13. Voskuyl AE, Zwinderman AH, Westedt ML, et al. Factors associated with the development of vasculitis in rheumatoid arthritis: results of a case-control study. *Ann Rheum Dis* 1996; 55:190–192.

14. Gordon DA. Deposition and storage diseases. In: Klippel JH, Weyand CM, Wortman RL, eds. *Primer on the rheumatic diseases.* Atlanta: Arthritis Foundation, 1997:329–330.

15. Achkar AA, Lie JT, Hunder GG, et al. How does previous corticosteroid treatment affect the biopsy findings in giant cell (temporal) arteritis? *Ann Intern Med* 1994;120:987–992.

16. Imbesi SG. Central nervous system vasculitis: Diffuse cerebral vasculitis with normal results on brain MR imaging. *AJR* 1999;173:1494–1496.

17. Cloft HJ, Phillips CD, Dix JE, et al. Correlation of angiography and MR imaging in cerebral vasculitis. *Acta Radiol* 1999; 40:83–87.

18. Wambach G, Finke K, Saborowski F. The clinical picture of panarteritis nodosa. *Med Klin* 1980;9,75:917–920.

19. Case records of the Massachusetts General Hospital. Weekly clinicopathological exercises. Case 38-1995. A 68-year-old man with paresthesias and severe pain in both hands [clinical conference]. *N Engl J Med* 1995;333:1625–1630.

20. Dawson DM. Entrapment neuropathies of the upper extremities [see comments]. *N Engl J Med* 1993;329:2013–2018.

21. Falk RH, Skinner M. The systemic amyloidoses: an overview. *Adv Intern Med* 2000;45:107–137.

22. Falk RH, Comenzo RL, Skinner M. The systemic amyloidoses [see comments]. *N Engl J Med* 1997;337:898–909.

23. Lightfoot RW, Jr., Michel BA, Bloch DA, et al. The American College of Rheumatology 1990 criteria for the classification of polyarteritis nodosa. *Arthritis Rheum* 1990;33:1088–1093.

24. Case records of the Massachusetts General Hospital. Weekly clinicopathological exercises. Case 18-1992. Asthma,

peripheral neuropathy, and eosinophilia in a 52-year-old man. *N Engl J Med* 1992;326:1204–1212.

25. Vaz RM, Formanek AG, Roach ES. Takayasu's arteritis. Protean manifestations. *J Adolesc Health Care* 1988;9:414–417.

26. Sack K. Monarthritis: differential diagnosis. *Am J Med* 1997; 102:30S–34S.

27. Braam B, Goldschmeding R, Derksen RH, et al. Clinical thinking and decision-making in practice. A patient with arthritis, skin lesions and a perforated nasal septum (see comments). *Ned Tijdschr Geneeskd.* 1999;143:1653–1658.

28. Anaya JM, Diethelm L, Ortiz LA, et al. Pulmonary involvement in rheumatoid arthritis. *Semin Arthritis Rheum* 1995;24: 242–254.

29. Gonzalez-Gay MA, Blanco R, Rodriguez-Valverde V, et al. Permanent visual loss and cerebrovascular accidents in giant cell arteritis: predictors and response to treatment [see comments]. *Arthritis Rheum* 1998;41:1497–1504.

30. Evans J, Hunder GG. The implications of recognizing large-vessel involvement in elderly patients with giant cell arteritis. *Curr Opin Rheumatol* 1997;9:37–40.

31. Case records of the Massachusetts General Hospital. Weekly clinicopathological exercises. Case 21-1979. *N Engl J Med* 1979;300:1204–1209.

32. Seo JW, Park IA, Yoon DH, et al. Thoracic aortic aneurysm associated with aortitis—case reports and histological review. *J Korean Med Sci* 1991;6:75–82.

33. Case 26-1985: Wegener's granulomatosis [Letter]. *N Engl J Med* 1985;313:1295.

34. Case records of the Massachusetts General Hospital. Weekly clinicopathological exercises. Case 26-1985. A 43-year-old woman with a progressive saddle-nose deformity. *N Engl J Med* 1985;312:1695–1703.

35. Mirzai R, Chang C, Greenspan A, et al. Avascular necrosis. *Compr Ther* 1998;24:251–255.

36. Salvarani C, Cantini F, Macchioni P, et al. Distal musculoskeletal manifestations in polymyalgia rheumatica: a prospective followup study [see comments]. *Arthritis Rheum* 1998;41:1221–1226.

37. Pouchot J, Sampalis JS, Beaudet F, et al. Adult Still's disease: manifestations, disease course, and outcome in 62 patients. *Medicine (Baltimore)* 1991;70:118–136.

38. Dalakas MC. Polymyositis, dermatomyositis and inclusion-body myositis [see comments]. *N Engl J Med* 1991;325: 1487–1498.

39. Sakane T, Takeno M, Suzuki N, et al. Behcet's disease. *N Engl J Med* 1999;341:1284–1291.

40. Rosenstein ED, Kramer N. Felty's and pseudo-Felty's syndromes. *Semin Arthritis Rheum* 1991;21:129–142.

41. Case records of the Massachusetts General Hospital. Weekly clinicopathological exercises. Case 20-1989. A 33-year-old woman with exertional dyspnea and Raynaud's phenomenon. *N Engl J Med* 1989;320:1333–1340.

42. Landry GJ, Edwards JM, McLafferty RB, et al. Long-term outcome of Raynaud's syndrome in a prospectively analyzed patient cohort. *J Vasc Surg* 1996;23:76–85.

43. ter Borg EJ, Piersma-Wichers G, Smit AJ, et al. Serial nailfold capillary microscopy in primary Raynaud's phenomenon and scleroderma. *Semin Arthritis Rheum* 1994;24:40–47.

44. Lin AN, Karasik A, Salit IE, et al. Group G streptococcal arthritis. *J Rheumatol* 1982;9:424–427.

45. Roberts-Thomson PJ, Rischmueller M, Kwiatek RA, et al. Rheumatic manifestations of infective endocarditis. *Rheumatol Int* 1992;12:61–63.

46. Felts WR. Ankylosing spondylitis: the challenge of early diagnosis. *Postgrad Med* 1982;72:184–193.

47. Case records of the Massachusetts General Hospital. Weekly clinicopathological exercises. Case 28-1998. A 64-year-old man with cranial-nerve palsies and a positive test for antinuclear cytoplasmic antibodies [clinical conference]. *N Engl J Med* 1998;339:755–763.

48. George TM, Cash JM, Farver C, et al. Mediastinal mass and hilar adenopathy: rare thoracic manifestations of Wegener's granulomatosis. *Arthritis Rheum* 1997;40:1992–1997.

49. Jones AC, Chuck AJ, Arie EA, et al. Diseases associated with calcium pyrophosphate deposition disease. *Semin Arthritis Rheum* 1992;22:188–202.

50. Hellmann DB. Spondyloarthropathy with hidradenitis suppurativa [clinical conference]. *JAMA* 1992;267:2363–2365.

51. Danjani AS, Bisno AL, Chung KJ, et al. Prevention of rheumatic fever. A statement for health professionals by the Committee on Rheumatic Fever, Endocarditis, and Kawasaki Disease of the Council on Cardiovascular Disease in the Young, the American Heart Association. *Circulation* 1988;78: 1082–1086.

52. Dougados M, van der LS, Juhlin R, et al. The European Spondylarthropathy Study Group preliminary criteria for the classification of spondylarthropathy [see comments]. *Arthritis Rheum* 1991;34:1218–1227.

53. Love LA, Leff RL, Fraser DD, et al. A new approach to the classification of idiopathic inflammatory myopathy: myositis-specific autoantibodies define useful homogeneous patient groups. *Medicine (Baltimore)* 1991;70:360–374.

54. Carroll GJ, Withers K, Bayliss CE. The prevalence of Raynaud's syndrome in rheumatoid arthritis. *Ann Rheum Dis* 1981;40:567–570.
55. Jones SM, Armas JB, Cohen MG, et al. Psoriatic arthritis: outcome of disease subsets and relationship of joint disease to nail and skin disease. *Br J Rheumatol* 1994;33:834–839.
56. Buskila D, Langevitz P, Gladman DD, et al. Patients with rheumatoid arthritis are more tender than those with psoriatic arthritis. *J Rheumatol* 1992;19:1115–1119.
57. Boulware DW, Schmid LD, Baron M. The fibromyalgia syndrome. Could you recognize and treat it? *Postgrad Med* 1990;87:211–214.
58. Hall S, Barr W, Lie JT, et al. Takayasu arteritis. A study of 32 North American patients. *Medicine (Baltimore)* 1985;64:89–99.
59. Wright V, Watkinson G. Articular complications of ulcerative colitis. *Am J Proctol* 1966;17:107–115.
60. Maksymowych WP, Chou CT, Russell AS. Matching prevalence of peripheral arthritis and acute anterior uveitis in individuals with ankylosing spondylitis. *Ann Rheum Dis* 1995;54:128–130.
61. Bulbul R, Williams WV, Schumacher HR, Jr. Psoriatic arthritis. Diverse and sometimes highly destructive. *Postgrad Med* 1995;97:97–6, 108.
62. Kafka SP, Condemi JJ, Marsh DO, et al. Mononeuritis multiplex and vasculitis. Association with anti-neutrophil cytoplasmic autoantibody [see comments]. *Arch Neurol* 1994;51: 565–568.
63. Neff AG, Greifenstein EM. Giant cell arteritis update. *Semin Ophthalmol* 1999;14:109–112.
64. Towheed TE, Hochberg MC. Acute monoarthritis: a practical approach to assessment and treatment. *Am Fam Physician* 1996;54:2239–2243.
65. Cherin P, Piette JC, Herson S, et al. Dermatomyositis and ovarian cancer: a report of 7 cases and literature review. *J Rheumatol* 1993;20:1897–1899.
66. Petri M. Infection in systemic lupus erythematosus. *Rheum Dis Clin North Am* 1998;24:423–456.
67. Harris MD, Siegel LB, Alloway JA. Gout and hyperuricemia [see comments]. *Am Fam Physician* 1999;59:925–934.
68. Agudelo CA, Wise CM. Gout and hyperuricemia. *Curr Opin Rheumatol* 1991;3:684–691.
69. Agnello V, Romain PL. Mixed cryoglobulinemia secondary to hepatitis C virus infection. *Rheum Dis Clin North Am* 1996; 22:1–21.

SUBJECT INDEX

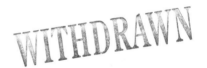